Y0-ACH-831

Health Counseling

by

MILTON SCHWEBEL, Ph.D.

Associate Professor in Education
Department of Guidance and Personnel Administration
New York University

and

ELLA FREAS HARRIS, M.D.

Assistant Professor in Education
Department of Physical Education, Health, and Recreation
Assistant University Physician, New York University

1951

CHARTWELL HOUSE, INC.

280 MADISON AVENUE NEW YORK, N. Y.

CHARTWELL HOUSE, INC.
280 Madison Avenue, New York, N. Y.

Printed in the United States of America

TO

BERNICE LOIS SCHWEBEL

AND

PIERSON PENROSE HARRIS

FOREWORD

The contents of this volume consider one of the most important problems in education: how can students be encouraged to improve their health behavior? Often we know what should be done to solve our health problems; too often we fail to put into action what we know. Methods are indicated through which teachers and counselors can assist others in recognizing their personal health problems, in understanding the necessity for action, in seeking professional advice, and in carrying out recommendations. Much emphasis is placed upon the need for client participation in the problem solution so that appropriate action will follow. The basic principles and illustrations from the authors' experiences are bound to be helpful in solving this problem.

This book makes a valuable contribution to the development of rational attitudes toward health and the subsequent improved living and increased productivity.

Morey R. Fields

PREFACE

This book has grown from our experience in teaching a course in health counseling at the School of Education, New York University, for five semesters. One of us was the instructor, the other the medical consultant.

This course was designed to add to the professional equipment of health workers. It sought to achieve this by helping health workers, and potential health workers, develop some awareness of their attitudes toward people, some understanding of the dynamics of the counseling relationship, and some skill in establishing this relationship. The course was also designed to sensitize other professional workers, such as counselors, teachers, social workers, and clergymen to the health problems and the counseling needs of their students and clients. In this course, we did not attempt to familiarize the student with the extensive research on counseling nor even with the variety of counseling orientations.

Some experienced counselors may question the wisdom of offering a single course in health counseling with the possible implication to the students that they will then be prepared to counsel. We do not pretend to make skilled counselors in one semester! We know, however, that with or without such a course in counseling, these health workers will be called on to perform the functions of the counselor. To deny this is to deny reality.

Some experienced health workers, grounded in the research methods of the physical sciences, may feel that the scientific tests of counseling are imperfect. Few counselors would deny that this criticism is justified. But to discard counseling attempts (and efforts to improve research design) until methods are perfected on a par with those used in the physical sciences is to cease helping humans until humans are as malleable as the objects of study of the physical sciences. This, of course, can never be. It is comforting to us, meanwhile, that the nondirective or client-centered counseling orientation, with which this book is most closely identified, has been responsible for the happy and prolific marriage of clinical practice (counseling) and experimental research.

We wish to express our gratitude to many of our colleagues on the faculty at New York University: to Professor Jay B. Nash, Chairman of the Department of Physical Education, Health, and Recreation, and Professor Robert Hoppock, Chairman of the Department of Guidance and Personnel Administration, for sharing with us their rich experience as authors, and for much understanding help during the months of writing; to Dr. John E. Sawhill, University Physician and Director of the Health Service, for his critical evaluation of chapters 8 and 9, and to Dr. J. Allison Montague, Psychiatrist in the University Health Service for critical review of chapters 8 and 10; to Professor William D. Wilkins, of the Department of Guidance and Personnel Administration, for his careful reading of the entire manuscript; to the Staff of the Health Service for creating the atmosphere that has made extensive health counseling possible; to our colleagues in our respective departments for encouragement; and to Miss Catherine Sista, our typist, for her forebearance at many a last-minute job.

Our thanks go also to Bernice L. Schwebel, second-grade teacher, for numerous suggestions on health counseling from her vantage point in education; to Professor Pierson P. Harris, of the English Department at Upsala College, for proofreading the entire manuscript; and to Dr. Walter Z. Schwebel, of Troy New York, for a pediatrician's reactions to the chapters on counseling.

Finally, our thanks to Professor Morey R. Fields, who in a busy life has managed to supply us with the necessary drive to "burn the midnight oil" more often than one would expect from authors of a book in *health* counseling!

Milton Schwebel
Ella F. Harris

TABLE OF CONTENTS

CHAPTER I

THE HEALTH COUNSELOR

Every activity of man involves his body to a lesser or greater degree. It is inescapable, therefore, that the body should be a factor in the problems that man faces.

Sometimes the ills of the body cause psychological problems. A defect, such as a paralyzed arm, can disturb the feelings of the individual to such an extent that he will not function efficiently. At other times the environment of the individual causes problems which produce certain bodily changes. Circumstances in the environment, such as rejection by his parents, can disturb the child so deeply that the normal functioning of his body is affected. Bodily symptoms, such as loss of appetite, may be obvious or they may be as subtle and unexpected as the breathing difficulties of the asthmatic.

Whether the disturbed bodily functioning is the cause or effect of his difficulties, the individual is in need of assistance. In school or on the job, both the individual and the institution benefit when the person in trouble is helped. Those who wish to help such persons must (1) understand themselves and the effect of their personalities on their clients, (2) know the dynamics of human behavior, including the relationship between bodily symptoms and emotional difficulties, and (3) possess a philosophy of counseling and the concomitant techniques. It does not matter what title the professional worker may bear. If he considers the helping of people in trouble his responsibility, he must understand behavior and be skilled in counseling. The need for this preparation becomes evident when we examine the experiences of an untrained person confronted with a counseling case.

Fred and His Home-Room Teacher

Fred, a seventeen year old junior in the academic curriculum in high school, is a better-than-average student. His written work is excellent, but his oral contributions are poor. He never volunteers to speak up during a discussion and, when called on by his teachers, he has difficulty expressing himself and appears to be tense and lacking in confidence. His home-room teacher feels that he is an unhappy boy.

The medical record indicates that he is in good health. He is of average height and weight for his age. His complexion is marred by acne eruptions.

Fred does not participate in any extracurricular activities. He appears to have no friends and he is rarely seen conversing with his classmates. He tends to remain in the background and to make no effort to change his behavior.

His mother told his home-room teacher at a PTA meeting:

> Fred has practically no friends. He goes to a movie about once a month with a boy of his age who lives nearby, but I have to push him to go out even then. Otherwise, he spends all his free time reading, working on his chemistry set, or listening to his records. He went to a few mixed parties, birthdays of teen-agers on the block, but he came home looking depressed. When I asked him why he felt that way, he said he was not interested in parties.

Disturbed by Fred's avoidance of social activity, his home-room teacher asked several of his subject teachers for their reactions to his behavior. Some of the opinions follow:

Fred is a bright boy who does good paper work, but is not so effective when he speaks. That's not objectionable. He is the scholarly research type. There is nothing wrong with that.

It is just a stage he is going through. Wait until he goes to college. He will blossom out.

He should do something about his acne. It is offensive. I imagine that is why he does not have friends. I wonder if his diet has been checked.

We should get him interested in clubs and sports. He needs friends. That's his trouble.

The home-room teacher favored the last two reactions and decided to use them as bases for helping Fred. She arranged an appointment with him during one of his free periods. She spent a full period with him on that day and the same time on another day in the following week.

The teacher reported on her experiences in a letter to a faculty member in a nearby college whose aid she requested. Following are excerpts from the letter:

I nearly talked myself hoarse, but the only change it brought about was in me; I found myself getting irritated. I reasoned with him, pleaded with him, presented all the facts, but I hardly stirred *him*. It's two months now and he seems completely unchanged.

When I suggested that he should go out with friends, he thanked me very politely. I could see, though, that he felt I was interfering in his affairs. He said to me, "I don't like having a lot of friends. I'd rather read, or work in my lab at home." I said that it was not healthy to be without friends, but he just answered, "My doctor says I'm in very good health." I told him I meant his mental health, and he stared at me coldly and said, "I'm not crazy, you know."

When I mentioned his acne, his face reddened and he said haltingly, "My family doctor . . . he takes care of it . . . I'm on a diet." I know he did not want me to talk about it.

By this time, I was angry with him. Now, in retrospect, I understand my anger. I was thwarted every way I turned. I wanted to help him, but I just couldn't. It seemed as if the very person I wanted to help was stopping me. I always thought that if you found out what was wrong with people and told them the facts, they would accept them and know what to do. But it didn't seem to work that way. He just threw the facts back in my face, so to speak, and made me feel helpless. I felt angry with him, but I was really angry with myself for failing so miserably. As a counselor, I'm a failure!

This teacher's experience was not unlike that of hundreds of others who have sincerely desired to help their students, colleagues, friends, patients, or employees. The chief instrument of counseling—the interview—appears to be so much like ordinary conversation that untrained beginners are frustrated when they find its appearance to be so deceiving.

Fred's home-room teacher was not the hopeless failure she may have felt herself to be. By her deeds she demonstrated that she had at least three characteristics of the good counselor:

(1) She was interested in Fred as a person, not simply as an academic machine that takes "subjects" and gets grades.

(2) She was able to recognize unhappiness in a boy whose behavior, characterized by silence in the classroom and good performance on written examinations, would be regarded by some teachers as most desirable in a student.

(3) She evaluated her interviews with Fred objectively even though the analysis disclosed her inadequacies as an interviewer.

Fred's teacher, a warm, friendly person, sensitive to the feelings of people, accepting her own limitations, has the potentialities of a good counselor. She has those personal qualities that are essential to successful counseling. Without them, no amount of training, no collection of techniques of interviewing, no advanced degrees will suffice to make one capable of serving people with adjustment problems. With them, one can learn the forces that "make us tick" (sometimes called the dynamics of behavior), one can learn the relationship between physical symptoms and emotional disturbance, one can develop a philosophy of counseling compatible with these dynamics and with one's philosophy of life, one can utilize techniques that grow naturally from this philosophy of counseling.

Fred's teacher can learn to counsel successfully. When she has learned, she will know why it is that talking one's self hoarse, reasoning, pleading, and presenting all the facts are not effective means of bringing about changes in the attitudes and the behavior of people with problems. Intelligent adults bite their fingernails. They know that they bite them. They know, too, that there are more attractive and efficient methods of trimming nails. Yet no amount of reasoning or cajolery will lead them to discontinue this practice. There are persons with physical beauty who regard themselves as unattractive, and others with high academic achievement who are distraught at their failure to attain grades implying perfection. Any attempt to be logical with them is almost as fruitless as the attempt to convince the schizophrenic (a psychotic or mentally ill person) that he is not dead when he insists that he is.[1]

Fred's teacher will learn that when she "preached" to him he experienced certain feelings that he did not share with her. When she suggested that he should go out with friends, Fred may have thought, "She thinks there's something wrong with me. Otherwise why would she try to make me change?" When she pointed out that it was not healthy to be friendless, perhaps he thought, "What's she getting at? What's wrong with me?" And finally when she indicated that she meant mental health, his reaction might well have been, "Just as I

[1] The inability of the maladjusted to deal rationally with their problems reflects in no way on the reasoning power of the human race. The emotionally disturbed can come to grips effectively with their environment when the counseling situation enables them to be objective with themselves and the world; the human race, given the same circumstances, can master the problems of nature and of social relationships.

thought. She thinks there's something wrong with me. She thinks I'm crazy!"

Fred's teacher tried to help, but she weakened her usefulness by arousing his suspicions and antagonisms. Instead of gaining his interest and confidence, she strengthened his defenses and made him, already an "island of self," even more impregnable to those who desired to help him. She did not know that what she is, what she does, what she says, and how she says it produce responses in Fred and in every other person with whom she has a relationship. To bring about a desirable change in Fred, she and every counselor working with every other Fred must know the effects of their personalities, their acts, their words, and their manner in order that these may facilitate rather than hinder the self-understanding and maturing of their clients.

Fred's teacher will learn to regard acne as one of the signals of possible maladjustment. For the adolescent who is experiencing powerful new urges driving him toward the opposite sex, the unattractive lesions of acne serve as a force, largely self-generated, which drives him away from this source of necessary satisfactions. Frustrated in the normal course of development, he must revert to other techniques to satisfy his needs. These other methods frequently exclude the necessary boy-girl relationships, and sometimes association with members of his own sex, and retard the social-emotional development of the adolescent.

It is this isolation of the individual, so common in many "health cases," that contributes to the making of that unfortunate adult who is mature in age, in physical structure, and in physiological functioning, but who is an adolescent in his skills of satisfying his needs for achievement, friendship, love, and sex.

Who Is a Health Counselor?

If young people are to be spared an unhappy adulthood, those who work with them must be trained to recognize the symptoms of immaturity. (In this book, only those symptoms are emphasized which are directly or indirectly related to health.) They must know how to establish a counseling relationship with the student-client; and how to proceed to that level of counseling which skill and time permit and the availability of "professional counseling" justifies. It may well be that the health counselor's function is simply that of creating an atmosphere in which the client will come to accept the desirability of referral to a specialist. This is no little service. It can be the difference between misery and happiness.

The health counselor, then, is a professional worker in human relations who helps individuals deal with problems of adjustment that involve illness, physical defect, or misconceptions about physiological processes.

He establishes the counseling relationship in interviews with motivated clients and he uses case work methods with the unmotivated.[2] His goal is to help them achieve more satisfying living; that is, living that is in greater harmony with objective reality. His minimum objective in those cases for which he lacks the skill or the time is referral to a specialist. When working with the motivated client, the counselor will help him recognize and accept the need for referral. With the unmotivated, the counselor attempts to reduce resistance to referral.

The term "health counselor" can well be applied to any member of the following groups:

(1) Those who are neither in professional counseling nor in the health field, but whose work brings them into contact with persons whose physical defects, illnesses, or poor health practices produce adjustment difficulties. This counseling group includes such professional workers as the classroom teacher, the clergyman, the athletic coach, and the recreation leader.

(2) Those professional health workers who are not trained

[2] The motivated client is one who comes voluntarily; the unmotivated person is one who does not recognize the need for counseling or who refuses counseling.

counselors or therapists, but who are called upon by circumstances to perform at least the screening and referral functions of health counseling. Persons in this category include physical educators, health educators, nurses, and physicians (other than psychiatrists).

(3) Those professional counselors and therapists who are not trained in health problems, but who work with some clients whose major problems are an outgrowth of physical defect or of illness, or whose emotional disturbances produce bodily symptoms. Examples of this type are the educational-vocational counselors in schools and community agencies and psychologists in schools, in child-guidance clinics, and in private practice.

The principles of counseling and of health are important in the work of each of these groups. The following section indicates the scope of this book in relation to these areas.

An Overview of the Book

The reader is interested in helping people. He wants to know how to help the student, patient, or client deal with his problems. There are some chapters in the book that will appear at first glance to be too theoretical and others that will seem to be proposing highly unrealistic and impractical methods of working with people. A few words now may avoid or minimize subsequent misunderstanding.

Some of the chapters are theoretical. That is, we have made *generalizations* based on observation of the behavior of *individuals*. The generalizations are built on the foundation of experiences of our students, clients, patients and acquaintances, not just on our own experiences and those of our families.

Theory rooted in experience is important because it enables man to control the concrete. We study the ways men learn in order to understand the process, to make generalizations about it, and thus to control and improve the learning experiences provided in our schools. We study the human body, make generalizations to be able to control and improve its condition. We observe the techniques of the very successful athletes, such as the Scandinavian runners, to analyze and understand their skill, to make generalizations that can be used in the training of other athletes.

We do not imply that the generalizations in this book are original. The theories of counseling indicated by us have been set up by philosophers, psychologists and social scientists from the early nineteenth century to the present. These theories are acceptable to us because they explain human behavior and the changes that go on in counseling, as we have experienced them, more adequately than any others. They will be acceptable to the reader only if they explain the phenomena of human behavior *as the reader experiences them*.

The authors are aware that much of the book is devoted to the explanation of a counseling approach that is effective only with a motivated person, that is, with the student who wants help. And many a reader will ask, "What about the students who don't know they have problems; or, if they do, don't want any help? What of a girl who needs corrective dental work but who refuses it? Do we leave it at that?"

The motivated person is no more important than the unmotivated. But the counseling relationship that makes for success with one is just as essential with the other. The philosophy that underlies the relationship of the counselor with the motivated student contains the principles of working with the unmotivated. Only the methods of dealing with the two are different.

The central theme of this book is as follows: From the earliest "learning," each of us begins to acquire meanings for the phenomena of our experience. Meanings become attached to mother, father, self, health, eating, sex, good boy (or girl), bad boy (or girl). When these meanings approximate objective reality, the person is "well-adjusted"; if there is a substantial discrepancy between meanings and reality, the individual is "poorly-adjusted." When a handicap, such as a loss of limb, means retribution to a person, his handicap may bring about so severe a feeling of guilt, self-deprecation, or sense of unworthiness that he becomes incapable of functioning effectively in any activity.

The goal of the counselor, whether in the area of health, vocational, or social problems, is to enable the client to change these meanings so that they more nearly approximate reality. Such a change alters behavior to be more in accord with the demands of life.

With the motivated client, these changes can be achieved through individual and group counseling. With the unmotivated client, the counselor must rely on the more cumbersome and less dependable case work approach, in which a study of the individual suggests appropriate manipulations of his physical and/or social environment.

What of the information-giving function of the counselor? A counselor is a resource person. He is not afraid to give information. However, there are several reservations to this statement. (1) He is aware that requests for information sometimes cloak problems that a client is too inhibited to present at the outset. He knows that if he acts as though his only function were to present information, the client might not raise his problem. (2) He is aware that the information he gives may be disturbing and is on the alert for its effects on the client, ready to perform his counseling function if necessary. (3) He does not have to know all that is known about health. (4) He does have to know the sources of such information. (5) His time is too valuable to be spent doling out information to individuals when this information is available from other sources, such as health education courses and literature written for the client's age group, that is, when the counselor is convinced that the client's request for information is not just his way of leading to a counseling problem.

In helping his clients, the health counselor plays a number of roles. He selects the role in accordance with the needs of the individual. With some people he functions largely as a counseling interviewer, with others as a case worker, and with still others as a resource person providing information.

His effectiveness depends in part on his skill in counseling and his knowledge of the principles of health, and in part on his ability to coordinate his efforts with the functions of other professional workers. For example, in the public high school, he will work with the physician in helping a student accept the limitations in activity demanded by a heart disease. He will work with the physical education department in helping the student accept a nonplaying role on a team, and with the director of the extracurricular program in helping the student find an outlet for his interests in clubs that do not make excessive demands. Of course, the counselor works with the teachers to interpret to them the difficulties of adjustment the student is facing and to gain their aid in the joint work of the health counseling team.

The health counselor recognizes that there are cases in which the time for counseling has passed. These are emergency situations involving acute physical and/or emotional illness for which there is no other recourse but immediate referral, without any attempt at establishing the counseling relationship.

Questions

1. What problems have you had in which you could have been helped by a counselor? By a health counselor? Do you have such problems now?
2. What problems have any of your acquaintances had in which they could have been helped by a health counselor?
3. How does your health status affect your social, educational, and vocational adjustment?
4. You have probably been interviewed at some time in your school or postschool life. What were the characteristics of the good interview and the good interviewer? Of the poor ones?
5. How would you have handled the case of Fred?

Bibliography

Arbuckle, Dugald S., *Teacher Counseling,* Cambridge: Addison-Wesley Press, 1950, p. 3-23. A clear statement on the need for and the role of counseling in the schools. The orientation of this book, in terms of counseling philosophy, is similar to ours.

Cowdry, E. V., *Problems of Ageing,* Baltimore: Williams & Wilkins Co., 1942. See chapter 28, "Psychological Aspects of Ageing," by Walter R. Miles and chapter 29, "Psychological Guidance for Older Persons," by George Lawton, on the changes that occur with aging and the need for counseling.

Davis, Frank G., *Pupil Personnel Service,* Scranton: The International Textbook Co., 1948. See chapters 6 and 7, "Pupil Personnel Service and Physical Well-Being," by John W. Rice, for description and incidence of ailments of students in the public schools.

Dunbar, Flanders, *Mind and Body: Psychosomatic Medicine,* New York: Random House, 1947. A nontechnical explanation of the interrelation of physical and psychological disturbances.

Leonard, M. L., *Health Counseling for Girls,* New York: A. S. Barnes, 1944.

National Education Association, Department of Classroom Teachers, *Fit to Teach,* Ninth Yearbook, 1938. Reports on a study which, among other findings, demonstrated a relationship between health and the quality of adjustment in the teaching profession.

Scott, Ira D., *Manual of Advisement and Guidance,* Washington: United States Government Printing Office, 1945. Principles and procedures in vocational counseling, especially with disabled clients.

Strang, Ruth M., and Dean F. Smiley, *The Role of the Teacher in Health Education,* New York: Macmillan, 1941. Chapters I-III for those who wish to become familiar with the needs for and foundations of health education, and Chapter IV for discussion of health problems prevalent in the schools.

Williamson, E. G., *How to Counsel Students,* New York: McGraw-Hill, 1939. See chapter 26, "Problems of Health and

Physical Disabilities," on the nature of health problems in schools and colleges and their significance in counseling. The counseling orientation of this author is very different from ours.

Chapter II

OBJECTIVES OF HEALTH COUNSELING

Counseling as an Aid to Learning

"Teachers teach! Why befuddle them with mental hygiene, child development, counseling, and all that sort of thing? What they really need to master is their teaching field."

This is not an uncommon remark even in this generation, a half-century after scientists demonstrated that the feelings of people were bound up with their efficiency in learning. Even among teachers, this view on the training and skills of the educator is unfortunately not rare, for there are some who believe that scholarship in one's field is sufficient to assure success and to serve the best interests of one's students. "Schools are for learning," they say, "and children who have mental trouble belong in an institution."

This attitude may reflect lack of training in the field of human behavior, or perhaps feelings of inadequacy in dealing with human problems. Regardless of the motives, however, the subject-matter-centered orientation of such teachers unavoidably denies their students the opportunity to work at maximum efficiency. Johnny who daydreams in class cannot make efficient use of the instructor's efforts, nor can he fulfill his potentialities. As long as the teacher's approach remains unchanged, Johnny's performance is likely to continue below capacity. Let this teacher ascribe his behavior to ineptness or just plain bad disposition, and let him, consistent with his philosophy, fail Johnny or demote him in grade. The cause of Johnny's daydreaming will not be eliminated; its incidence may even be increased. The waste of the instructor's effort and of Johnny's potentialities continues.

Such a teacher is not aware that among the thousand students in his school, very few are in need of care in a mental institution while many could appreciably improve their academic performance (and general adjustment) with the aid of a teacher sensitive to their needs and capable of satisfying some of these needs by means of the curriculum.

A second type of teacher says: "Of course we can no longer concentrate on our subject matter alone. The belief that the scholar can walk into the classroom and transfer his knowledge to the brains of his students, as if by a funnel inserted in the ears, is now discredited and antiquated. Besides mastering his teaching field, the teacher of today must understand human behavior. He must know why the students seem to act so irrationally at times. But beyond this point, he should not and need not go. He does not have to learn how to counsel. That is the specialist's job."

The third type of teacher goes one step farther: "Understanding of our students, yes, indeed! But to understand them is not enough. They need help. Let's be realistic. Where are all the specialists? Few as they are in proportion to the demand in the metropolitan areas, they are almost nonexistent in the rural sections of the country. Must our youngsters go unaided? I say no! If we can learn how to teach them comparatively meaningless facts about dead people and faraway places, surely we can learn the skills to teach them meaningful facts about themselves and their world, skills like counseling with individuals and groups."

The difference between the first and third teacher is no less than a difference in the philosophy of education and the psychology of learning under which each operates. To the first teacher, education is primarily concerned with knowledge which happens incidentally to be transmitted by people. To the third teacher, education is concerned with people who learn in the process of satisfying their needs.

According to the best representatives of the first type, facts are transmitted successfully by reliance on external motivators, such as a stimulating lecture, desire for success in the course or for recognition in the class. According to the best representatives of the third type, learning proceeds successfully when the student becomes aware of his needs and recognizes the roles of student, teacher, and curriculum in satisfying those needs. To the first teacher, education is something that happens to an individual, something external added to him. To the third teacher, education is a process of growth flowing from the interaction of individual and environment; it is a process of change within him.

The personal life of the student can facilitate or obstruct the process of learning. The young adolescent who is confident in the security of his home life can be expected to function effectively in school. His classmate who has been shaken by discord in the home and works in the shadow of divorce and a broken home cannot be expected to perform well. There is no disagreement in respect to this principle of learning. Even our first teacher, quoted in the opening paragraph of the chapter, would not take issue with it. Disagreement occurs only when implementation of the principle is discussed, for—as we have already indicated—some educators believe that the school must studiously avoid involvement in the personal, emotional problems of their students. They will assume the responsibility for referring them to specialists, but no more than that.

This practice may be justified in dealing with the relatively small number of students who are psychotic or prepsychotic. But at which point in a listing of emotional disturbances from psychotic to "near-normal" is the school to assume responsibility? For example, is the daydreamer who misses much of the classroom work to be referred to a specialist? Or is the school going to aid him? Is he to be denied any aid and permitted only to remain in class, working at a low level of efficiency? What do we do with the following individuals: the young girl disturbed by the physiological changes of puberty; the college student who cannot reconcile his moral training, his pressing needs, and the temptations of a life fraught with new freedoms; the young adult, an arrested tuberculosis patient, caught between the conflicting health needs for a short work-week and the job-market demands for an unhandicapped worker?

If we do not help these young people, we must anticipate that for a large percentage of them, there will be a discrepancy between capacity and achievement. Their need for help is nowhere more starkly drawn than in the attrition reports of colleges with highly selective standards for admission. In 276 such institutions, where students are selected in large numbers on the basis of their academic ability, the loss of students due to academic failure ranged from 37% in men's colleges with enrollment exceeding 1,000, to 61% in coeducational institutions with more than 1,000 students. "In colleges such as Dartmouth and other New England colleges which are very selective in admissions, almost no one fails because of lack of ability. Failures result from lack of interest, misdirected energy, inability to adjust to freedom from home or equivalent supervision, and temperament." [1]

A nation that permits such human waste cannot remain healthy. A country that points with pride to its measures for over half a century to conserve its physical resources can ill afford the erosion of the roots of human talent. Counseling is one means of conserving our great resources. There are other means, some of them more fundamental than counseling. A radical change in the need of parents to satisfy their sense of possessiveness in the dependency of their children would make for healthier, better-adjusted citizens of to-

[1] Archibald MacIntosh, *Behind the Academic Curtain,* New York: Harper and Brothers, 1948, p. 62.

morrow. Basic changes in our attitudes toward anatomy and physiology that might permit wholesome discussion of the sexual functions of the body and healthy assumption of adult sex roles would eliminate one cause of adjustment problems and reduce the need for counseling. A full-employment economy, unthreatened by impending depression, would eliminate the anxieties of unemployment, including those that make for many maladjustments, and would modify the high job specifications of an oversupplied labor market that discriminates against the handicapped. A society at peace with itself and the world, unthreatened by impending war, would eliminate the anxieties of family separation, atomic destruction, and premature death. Counseling does not occur in a vacuum and the counselor cannot ignore the dominant influences of culture in shaping personality. In this book, however, we concentrate on counseling as a method of human conservation, though conscious of the fact that many of the problems with which we deal are socially produced and socially eradicable.

Schools have no monopoly on counseling. If the discussions in this book seem largely cloaked in educational terminology, it should be noted that all significant professional relationships with people require learning for their successful consummation with consequent change in behavior. This is obvious in the case of the public-health nurse who teaches the young mother sanitary methods of preparing food for her new baby. It is not so obvious in the case of the physician who diagnoses symptoms of heart disease and informs the patient that he must discontinue participation in competitive sports. Surely, the efforts of both nurse and physician will have been in vain unless the young mother applies the sanitary methods and the patient adopts the new patterns prescribed by the physician. Unless the "teachings" of the nurse and the physician are translated by their "students" into behavior changes, they have been no more effective than the teaching of a classroom instructor of grammar whose students cannot write an intelligible sentence, or of the safety instructor whose students cross the street against the traffic signal. Whenever the objective of a professional relationship is the learning of something new and a change in behavior, the professional person can contribute to his effectiveness by understanding the dynamics of behavior and the techniques of controlling them through counseling.

Special Counseling Needs of the Handicapped

The Constitution with its Bill of Rights was written for all of the people of the United States. The lame, the halt, the blind, and all those whose physical and mental defects have set them apart in appearance, in behavior, or in productive capacity were not denied the privileges or the obligations of citizenship in that document. Yet, circumstances have come to set them apart from the rest of the population, and this isolation has been deepened by its effects on their perception of their place in the world. They suffer a sociological and a psychological detachment. It is fruitless to attempt to establish in any particular case which was cause and which effect; whether the psychological effect of amputation produced the social withdrawal of the client, or whether rejection by society, as represented by a member of the opposite sex or by an employer, produced the psychological concomitants of withdrawal. In either event, the amputee needs help. A counselor cannot change the attitudes of the persons with whom his client associates and surely not of those who pass him by on the street, staring fixedly at the hook projecting from a sleeve, or at a hobbled walk. But he can help his client understand his own feelings toward these people and develop a positive outlook on life built on the realities of his *self* and of the culture of which he is a part.

Counseling has been proposed as a method of correcting maladjustment and of facilitating learning in the general population. The same conditions that impair the effectiveness of the normal or unhandicapped population apply equally to the ill or handicapped population. For the handicapped, however, there are additional obstructions. The high-school freshman whose parents have browbeaten him into silence and submission has difficulty enough in satisfying his needs for achievement and status, for feeling that he "belongs." Whether or not he has other limitations, here is already serious cause for unhappiness and underachievement. The chronically ill and the handicapped are susceptible to all of the disrupting influences that affect the general population. In addition, they must counter the deterring circumstances of their ailment. Already pressed for survival as a social being, our browbeaten boy would take further beating, if the aftereffects of rheumatic fever prevented his participation in competitive sports. Even a minor ailment, such as acne eruptions on his face, would aggravate this boy's social problems and further complicate the tasks of the counselor.

The health counselor has been defined as an individual who assists people in dealing with adjustment problems, stemming from illness, physical defect, or ignorance of physiological processes. The skills of the counselor are invaluable in working with clients from the so-called "normal" population who have such problems; these skills are *indispensable* if we are to achieve success with that heterogeneous group of chronically ill and handicapped persons whose problems are doubly compounded.

The Limitations of Counseling

Counseling is not a panacea. Counselors do not perform miracles. They simply provide the client with an opportunity to see himself and his world more clearly, more objectively. They cannot enable him to see what is not there. They cannot make a plain face beautiful, nor can they transform a stump into an arm. They cannot stop the teen-agers in their cruel teasing of one of their group who is bald from the effect of a fever, nor can they change the attitudes of employers toward the physically handicapped.[2,3] In short, counseling will not produce changes in social values that make the loss of arm or hair, or the plainness of face so incalculably painful to the individual concerned. It can only help him to sharpen his focus so that he can look beyond his limitation and see the positive factor, the strength and the hope that are latent within all of us and without which no man can live.

The educational/vocational counselor can neither increase the number of jobs nor alter the pattern of demand so that more places are available in the attractive professions. The counselor can only assist the individual in choosing the educational and vocational objectives that best suit him and in recognizing the factors that support and those that oppose the possibility of success. If in the course of counseling, the client has developed skills in coping with problems, he will be better able to deal with the barriers to satisfying his needs.

Health counseling, as any other counseling, does not seek to and is not capable of changing social conditions and social values. Its aim is much more modest: to provide the counselee with the opportunity to view his piece of world (his self, family, friends, his sex role, his spiritual, social and political

[2] "Employer relations representatives can play a big part in the selective placement program by helping to overcome employer resistance. This resistance of employers is a remnant of primitive times when the handicapped were forced out of the tribe or clan or even worse. The prejudice is still with us and most of the time it is unreasonable." This excerpt is from the article, "A Manager's View of Selective Placement," by Roy V. Stewart in *Employment Security Review* 17 (September 1950) 11-13. The entire issue of this journal was devoted to placement of the handicapped, under the title of "A Decade of Selective Placement."

[3] Muriel Jennings, "The Need for Employer Education as Regards the Abilities of the Physically Impaired Worker." Publication pending. A summary by the author follows: "By interview of about twenty employers in New York in a manner designed not to reveal the biases of the investigator, the following were revealed: (1) A tremendous gap exists between the theories and ideals the employer professes as regards employment of the physically disabled, and his actual practices; and (2) this sampling of employers held as truths many false beliefs and misconceptions pertaining to the production efficiency, the rate of absenteeism, and accident proneness of the physically disabled."

values) in the free, permissive atmosphere that makes for objectivity. Objectivity, the recognition of positive as well as negative forces, provides for mature decision and action.

It is advisable to recognize these limitations at the outset. The great strides in counseling during the past 75 years have been made by clinicians who have subjected hypotheses to the rigorous scrutiny of scientific tests. In some of these tests experimental controls have been introduced, such as the studies of Rogers[4] and his colleagues, whereas in others the judgment and creativity of a great mind like Freud's[5] have been used. Despite abuses and claims sometimes in excess of the actual data, the past contributions have had the mark of the scientific discipline. The student of counseling would do well to follow this tradition, recognizing limitations, avoiding extravagant claims, and attributing to counseling no more than the findings of science and the skill of the counselor justify.

Specific Objectives of Health Counseling

We have developed the theme that counseling is invaluable in improving the effectiveness of many students, workers, and patients, and that persons who are ill or handicapped are compelled to make adjustments beyond those made by the general population. The over-all objective of counseling is clearly to help clients with their problems or, stated differently, to assist them in developing or improving techniques of need-satisfaction consistent with themselves. This broad statement is subject to so many different interpretations that it demands further spelling out. The following specific objectives are intended for that purpose.

(1) **Acceptance of self.** Whatever the approach of the counselor, one of the goals essential for the culmination of success of counseling is the client's self-acceptance. This term does

[4] Carl R. Rogers, *Client Centered Therapy,* New York: Houghton Mifflin, 1951.

[5] Sigmund Freud, *New Introductory Lectures on Psycho-Analysis,* New York: W. W. Norton and Co., 1933.

not imply a state of resignation on the part of the client; it does not mean that he accepts as immutable and irrevocable the limitations of skill, knowledge, or even personality that he now possesses. Self-acceptance is not meant to *freeze* each individual at his present status, making growth, change, and improvement incompatible with counseling. On the contrary, self-acceptance, the objective appraisal of self, is intended to free the person from the restraints of self-depreciation and from the equally handicapping effects of self-aggrandizement.

The concept of self-acceptance means recognition of what constitutes one's self, such as perception of one's traits, characteristics, and abilities, consistent with those made by others less involved emotionally. Realistic appraisal of self is essential for efficient living, for the maintenance of good health. The distorted self-concept in its most extreme form is found in the delusion of the psychotic. He pictures himself as, and lives out the role of, a king, a saint, or a criminal. There are reasons for such perceptions of self which will be discussed later; what is of significance at this point is the fact that behavior is an outgrowth of the manner in which one sees one's self and one's world. The psychotic who regards himself as Napoleon will behave in an aggressive, domineering, dictatorial fashion. The patient who regards himself as evil and sinful will withdraw into a shell, fearful and craven, waiting for the avenging blow of an omniscient power.

What has this to do with the "average" individual whom we meet in the school, the hospital, the physician's office, the recreation rooms of community center or church? This principle applies to them also: behavior is a product of the self concept, of the way one sees oneself. Only when there is a great discrepancy between the picture one has of oneself and the realities of one's ability, do we find problems like these:

> High school sophomore, I. Q. 98, grades of C and D in mathematics and science; occupational objective: physician.
>
> College freshman, female, beautiful face, shapely figure,

avoids the company of men because she feels she is unattractive.

High school student whose physical condition prohibits competitive activity avoids the company of boys "because they think I'm a sissy."

Well educated man of forty-five, bachelor, plays basketball, dates girls of twenty, because he thinks he is "still a young man."

Young wife who says that she wants children but who refuses to have any, because if her children were to have a choice of entering "this sinful, hateful world" they would reject it.

In working with the first client, the counselor knows that the high school sophomore will suffer frustrations and will not experience the success one needs for happy, satisfying living until his curricular choice, and his occupational plans are in closer alignment with his capacity. Such changes are meaningless when they are wrought by compulsion. The student himself must come to see that he is unfit for the profession he has selected, for only then can he begin to find means of satisfying his needs, such as that for status, which are compatible with his talents. Our high school sophomore says during a counseling session:

Student: Maybe I'm just fooling myself. I can't seem to get this geometry. It keeps on getting worse and I'm falling behind all the time. Maybe I'm just not meant for it.

Counselor: It's just getting you down, and you're beginning to wonder if you should be taking it.

Student: Why should I break my head over something I'm no good at? I guess I'm just not cut out for deep studying.—If I can't go to college I won't. My Pop never went—he didn't even finish high school—and he gets along.

The counseling does not end at this point. When the client is able to accept himself as he is, with his limitations, his physical defects, and any other irremediable encumbrances, then he is ready to make plans that can be fulfilled and thus give him satisfactions. We turn now to the second specific objective.

(2) **Solving the problem at hand.** Now the client is ready to plan realistically. He has gone through the process of discovering himself and of realizing that he can live with this self. He has laid the cards on the table and found them satisfying. It is as if he were saying to the world: "This is me, and I can live with me! I'm O.K. this way; I can get along." He begins to plan for the use of his powers. Now he is prepared to carry into action whatever changes in behavior are necessary to make life something more than tolerable. He seeks to effect those changes that will permit him to attain need-satisfaction. An excerpt from another interview with our high school sophomore illustrates the achievement of this specific objective in counseling.

> *Student:* You remember the things we were talking about last week. You know,—about college not being everything? Well, I talked with my mother about the same thing the other day, and the funny thing about it—she sorta felt the same way!
>
> *Counselor:* You were really surprised.
>
> *Student:* I thought she was going to start talking about the fella next door. He's going to the State University and he's going to be a lawyer. My mother used to talk about the money he'd make. But I see now you can do pretty well if you're a mechanic or a machinist. You know, I read some of those little books in the library—the ones you told me about —and I'd like to talk about how I can try myself out for that work. I think I'd like it.

This boy has discovered that he can accept himself as a person lacking the ability for success as a physician without losing the love and support of his mother. He has found other fields that appear to offer him the opportunity for success and the satisfaction of adolescent and adult needs.

Following are excerpts taken from several interviews with a veteran of World War II, a college freshman, Peter, age 23, whose right arm was amputated below the elbow, and who wears an orthopedic hook.

First Interview

Peter: Why should anyone be interested in me? No girl wants to dance with a hook around her waist. They turn white when they feel it.

Counselor: You feel your hook drives people away from you.

Peter: Well, it's not just the hook. It's me. The hook is part of me now and even without it I'd be just as much a . . . well, a freak.

Counselor: You see yourself as a freak.

Peter: And who wants to go with a freak. It's not just the women either. The fellows too, but somehow that doesn't bother me so much. But I know what they're thinking. They're like the people who stare at me on the bus. "Poor guy. What an awful thing. I pity him. We should all be good to him." I *hate* that.

Counselor: You feel that people are interested in you just out of pity and it burns you up.

Fourth Interview (one month later)

Peter: Funny thing happened the other night. Supposing I tell you about it.

Counselor: Sure. Go ahead, Pete.

Peter: I think I told you that I'm rooming with Tony. . . . Well, we had an argument the other night. The first time. (Pauses and smiles.)

Counselor (also smiling): You seem to have gotten quite a kick out of it!

Peter: Tony wanted me to go to a party with him in town. I said no and he called me a mule and it really got hot for a while. Then I said "dammit, don't kill me with pity" and when I said it I felt as if I were hitting him with something.

Counselor: It seemed like a way of getting back at him for something.

Peter: Yeh, as if I was just jealous because he did the things I wanted to. He got angry and called me plenty and told me to rot in my sack if I wanted to. And you know this was the first time I felt that he really liked me for myself.

Seventh Interview

Peter: Tony took me to a party Saturday night. Reminded me of . . . (talks of last party he had attended, on a leave to Paris in November, 1944.). . . . At first I didn't like it. I started feeling sorry for myself.

Counselor: Feeling sorry for yourself got in your way.

Peter: Yeh. It seemed as if I was all hooks, as if that was all anyone could see. And all I did was try to hide it when I danced with one girl. I kept thinking, can she see it? What will she say? And I forgot her name and couldn't even carry on a conversation.

Counselor: You were thinking so much about yourself that you couldn't pay attention to the girl.

Peter: That was just it. Well, Tony saw it too, and he came over and made a crack about the girl and me. At first I got angry but then I just laughed.

Counselor: You mean what you had been doing seemed funny to you?

Peter: Well, something like that. Everything we'd been talking about seemed to hit home and the hook didn't seem so important any more.

Counselor: You began to see things in a different way.

Peter: Yeh, and to show you what happened (red faced and beaming) I've got a date Saturday night.

(3) Skill in handling future problems. A counselor interested in the welfare of his client hopes that the time and effort devoted to the process will do more than aid in solving the present problem. He makes of the counseling sessions a learning situation so that the client will develop skills in appraising himself and his environment "objectively." In addition the client will become familiar with the resources of the community and will learn to make decisions in a mature fashion. This knowledge and these skills are then available for use whenever the client is confronted with new problems. Like the good businessman, the counselor creates such relationships with his "customer" to make him willing to return when the need arises. Unlike the businessman, the counselor seeks to do his job in such a way that his client will have no need to return.

Questions

1. Reconstruct Peter's self-concept from the contents of the first interview.
2. Reconstruct his self-concept from the seventh interview.
3. How did his attitude toward himself affect his behavior?
4. What brought about the change?
5. What change would have been produced had the counselor told Peter during the first interview not to concentrate so much on his hook, and to socialize more?
6. What is your self-concept?
7. How did it develop?
8. Are there any aspects of your self that have changed? How did this occur?
9. Are there any aspects of your self that you have wanted to change but you have not succeeded in changing? What methods have you used? Why did they fail?

Bibliography

Barker, Roger G., Beatrice A. Wright, and Mollie R. Gonick, *Adjustment to Physical Handicap and Illness: A Survey of the Social Psychology of Physique and Disability,* New York: Social Science Research Council, 1946. See chapter 7, "Employment of the Disabled." This book contains a bibliography on each of the disabilities.

Rogers, Carl R., *Counseling and Psychotherapy,* New York: Houghton Mifflin Co., 1942. Although the point of view of the author has been revised on the basis of new experience and is reported in the volume listed next, this is still one of the clearest expositions of concepts in counseling. See chapter 1 on the use of counseling in various institutions.

Rogers, Carl R., *Client-Centered Therapy,* New York: Houghton Mifflin Co., 1951.

Williamson, E. G., *Counseling Adolescents,* New York: McGraw-Hill, 1950. See chapters 1 and 2 and p. 51 to 54 on the place of counseling in education and the role of the counselor.

Chapter III

A PHILOSOPHY OF HEALTH COUNSELING

Philosophy is an awesome word. To the student it frequently conveys the image of a cloistered pedant creating complex systems that are chiefly characterized by their unrelatedness to everyday life. Such a distorted concept is the logical sequence of reading books and hearing lectures on the ideology of the philosopher presented out of context with the social, economic, and political dynamics of the society in which he lived. The values and attitudes of the philosopher, no less than of the client and his counselor, are a product of his life in a social environment. The student can comprehend the meaning and appreciate the significance of a philosophical system only in terms of its social context.

Philosophy is defined as the study and knowledge of the principles that cause, control, or explain facts and events.[1] The facts and events of one culture in the eighteenth century are not the same as those of our culture in the twentieth century.

The philosopher does no more than attempt to explain the phenomena of his world; to establish principles that underlie personal, social, and physical behavior so that man and his society may be better equipped to control this behavior. The scientist who is a philosopher employing dif-

[1] *The Winston Dictionary,* Philadelphia: The John C. Winston Co., 1944.

ferent techniques of validating his hypotheses seeks the same objectives. Both are limited in their efforts by the boundaries of their experience; they cannot go beyond. In other words, they cannot see beyond their own horizons. The theories set forth by philosopher or scientist are a function of their field of perception. Examining the phenomena of his society or of the physical world, the scientist abstracts the basic principles that explain them. This is not to say that there can be no progress, that society cannot develop beyond the limits of perception of its philosophers. The explanatory principles then permit a control over behavior that makes for changes in the physical or social world, leading to new perceptions and changes in theory and practice.

If the counselor is to be efficient, he must determine the principles that explain human behavior. He cannot aid his clients in changing their behavior unless he understands the dynamic forces that control it. There is no bag of tricks, no set of techniques, no secret formulas that will substitute for a philosophy of counseling.

The fact is that all counselors, like all people, operate on the basis of a set of principles whether or not they are aware of this. The person who verbally lashes a child for his repeated failure to do his homework assumes that such action will favorably alter the child's behavior. Approaches like the following make the same assumption, but each is obviously based on different principles: keep the child after school; send a note to the parents predicting the child's failure; tell the child that such action will lead to failure; examine his records and discuss them with other staff members.

All counselors operate on the basis of certain principles. Whether or not designed for such purpose, their counseling techniques imply that humans behave in certain fashions. The counselors work is most effective when those principles are accurate reflections of reality. The counselor who seeks to change his client's behavior by threatening him with reprisals is as ineffective and as outmoded as the navigator charting a course in terms of fifteenth century principles of astronomy.

We seek in this chapter to assist in formulating a philosophy of counseling based on principles of human behavior. This is only one of several philosophies that are currently accepted. While it is well for the counselor to be familiar with all the approaches, he can operate in terms of only one of them even if he intellectually espouses eclecticism. Either he does or he does not believe that counseling must be firmly rooted in a respect for the dignity of each individual. He cannot believe both, and his methods will reflect his sincere belief more accurately than his verbalization of it. Similarly, the counselor does or does not believe that fundamental changes in behavior can occur only when the client has the need within himself to make such changes, or only when the changes are self-motivated. He cannot believe both simultaneously. He might be capricious, his views changing frequently, but, even in this case, the other techniques he employs are in direct relation with his beliefs.

Since counseling techniques are a function of a counseling philosophy, that philosophy should be clearly understood, meaningful and acceptable to the counselor. He then has a constant base line for evaluation of his professional work. He can check the appropriateness of his responses, his plans, his staff discussions, his utilization of resources in terms of understanding the dynamics of behavior. The counselor—as scientist—seeks to validate his effectiveness by determining criteria of counseling success and then determining the degree to which his completed cases measure up to these criteria, such as: are the clients' marriages successful; are they adjusting on their jobs? This difficult and long-term evaluation is essential for the further development of counseling. The counselor—as practitioner—works with clients who cannot wait for these answers. He must rely on a check of consistency between his practices and his interpretation of human behavior, with the only possible empirical verification being his judgment of desirable change in the client's adjustment.

A philosophy of counseling is not a formula. It cannot be learned by repetition and review as one learns the spelling of words. It must be believed, and to be believed it must be acceptable to the individual. One cannot believe in a counseling approach that emphasizes permissiveness if one cannot accept the values and the behavior of the client, whatever they are. Nor can one foster independence and self-direction in a client if one cannot accept decisions made by others. There are some for whom the philosophy presented in this chapter is unacceptable and therefore unworkable. Some among them may lack the personal qualities for counseling; others may find themselves more suited to another philosophy. The personal characteristics appropriate to the approach described here will be discussed in the next chapter.

Two Basic Assumptions

In his quest for knowledge, man has sought for a unifying principle that would suffice to explain phenomena. He has not been content with understanding the forces that produce response in the ameba. What principles, he has asked himself, explain the behavior of all unicellular organisms, of reptiles, of birds, of mammals? Are there underlying principles that explain the behavior of all of them? Is there *one* basic principle?

This movement in the direction of fundamental principle has characterized the history of science. The fruitful life of Albert Einstein has been dedicated to the task of discovering a basic theory that would explain the behavior of subatomic particles as well as that of the stars and planets.

The psychologist likewise seeks a hypothesis that will explain the behavior of all people under all circumstances. It must apply equally to normal, neurotic, and psychotic; to infant girl and senile man; to Negro, White, and Yellow; to American, Russian and Chinese.

Our philosophy of counseling is hypothetical; it has not been verified. It is presented here in the form of two basic assumptions both of which have an abundance of data to support them, but neither of which has been better established than assumptions made by other systems of counseling. No group of counselors can claim conclusive evidence in support of its position. Psychological science has not yet developed the precise and unqualified tests of its hypotheses that Einstein was able to employ in verifying his theory of relativity.

Although our counseling approach is founded on assumptions, they appear to be well grounded in scientific data. What is more, the second assumption constitutes a unifying principle that presumably explains all human behavior and thus represents an advance in psychological science.

The first assumption is the existence of a drive for growth, health, and maturity.

Scientists have greatly enriched our knowledge of the behavior of the human being during his prenatal and his infant life. They have recorded in detail a sequence of events that follow conception—among them the appearance of the first behavior response—a reflex act of the fetus early in the third month of life in the uterus. Yet we are lacking in precise information on the functional level of the psychological equipment at birth. The following questions cannot be answered with assurance: "Is the infant born with a personality? Does he have at birth the potentialities for neurosis, psychosis, or normality? Did he learn while in the uterus and does he have memory of that learning, if any, or evidence of any racially inherited, deep-seated primitive instincts?"

Unfortunately scientists have been unable to investigate these questions directly. Inferences from research that borders on these problems would suggest a negative answer to each of these questions. *Tabula rasa,* or clean slate, as Descartes, French mathematician and philosopher of the seventeenth century, described the mental condition of man at birth, appears to be an apt and accurate description of today. The infant has sensory organs ready to operate shortly after birth, but he has neither knowledge nor attitudes. He has potentialities for a certain quality of performance and for physical attractiveness, both of which are significant in the development of personality, but he has no personality. He can respond to only a limited number of stimuli, and his unlearned responses to these are not unique. He has not yet "learned" or acquired that distinctness of response that is called personality.

There does appear to be in all human beings a drive for life, health, growth, and maturity. The reflexes of the infant are designed to preserve life: He cries when he is in pain, whether the pain is due to lack of food, digestive difficulties, the prick of an open pin, high body temperature, or low atmospheric temperature; he blinks when something comes too close to his eyes; he swallows when food reaches his mouth. As he grows older, and is given a choice of a wide variety of foods in the so-called cafeteria-feeding experiments,[2] he selects those that make him thrive, rejecting some foods on which other children thrive. This behavior is not learned; it is inherent in the organism. This "wisdom of the body" as one investigator[3] called it is directed toward its survival and growth, toward the satisfaction of the needs of the organism.

As the child grows, he learns new methods of satisfying his needs. When he is hungry now, he does not cry; he asks for food. He has learned another, a more mature method of communication. The utilization of mature skills increases the effectiveness of need-satisfaction. There is nothing mysterious about this characteristic. As he experiences the unfolding of greater intellectual and physical prowess, the young human

[2] C. M. Davis, "Self-Selection of Diet by Newly Weaned Infants," *American Journal of Children*, 36, 651-679 (1928). The influence of oversolicitous and overbearing parents is not permitted to influence the food choices of the infants and children in these experiments.

[3] Walter B. Cannon, *The Wisdom of the Body*, New York: W. W. Norton and Co., 1939.

being recognizes and employs improved techniques of operation. He learns how to set one block squarely on another so that his "house" will not come crashing to the floor; he learns how to enunciate more clearly so that the candy clerk will give him what *he* wants; he learns the power of a smile and the value *for himself* of cooperation with others. These positive changes are regarded as marks of maturity and they come about seemingly because the individual is motivated by self-interest.

Without need to resort to an esoteric interpretation or to attribute it to a supernatural power, this drive for life, growth, health, and maturity can be regarded as a characteristic of living matter, whether of the protozoon or of the complex human organism. All animals attempt to preserve themselves. Whether by reflex act, by instinct, or by learning (it is not easy to determine where the second ends and the third begins), they attempt to defend themselves against the ravages of nature. Sometimes their structure is such that they fail in their attempts and become extinct as, for example, the dinosaur; or the methods they adopt to defend themselves and to satisfy their needs create severe problems, as with the alcoholic. This in no way contradicts the basic assumption that the underlying purpose of behavior is to preserve life and health and to permit the development of the organism and the attainment of its maturity, that is, the unfolding of those personal and social skills and attitudes which are conducive to the most efficient satisfaction of needs.

The second assumption *postulates that the basic need of all persons is maintenance and enhancement of "the self."*

What motivates the drive for life, growth, health, and maturity? What leads the individual to learn the many and variegated skills and attitudes that give him a mastery over his environment? What single force drives on all persons, no matter at what point on the continuum of "normality"—the energetic child and the enervated senile adult, the healthy, happy young adult and his neighbor of the same age, a schizophrenic living out his days in a fantasied community peopled by creations of his imagination?

All persons possess a drive for life, growth, health, and maturity, because this drive satisfies their basic need for the maintenance and the enhancement of the self. "Maintenance of self" means more than just the preservation of the body. The "self" embraces much more than the protoplasm that constitutes it, much more even than the configuration of the protoplasm that makes each person's body, including his face, unique. The self includes those attitudes, values, goals, affiliations which compose the "what I am" of an individual. For *all* persons, "self" is more than the body; self is "I," and it is the maintenance and enhancement of this self that is man's basic need.

Let us postulate that among our readers are seniors majoring in health education who have some of the following characteristics:

They believe they have better-than-average intelligence and are capable of completing the requirements for a degree.

They believe they are good teachers.

They feel that they are attractive.

They feel that they are liked.

These people treasure life. The continued survival and efficient operation of their bodies are important, and how terrible would be the blow to learn that they had an illness that would produce marked disability or limitation. They also treasure the other aspects of self, the feelings they have of their abilities, and how terrible would be the blow to learn that they did not possess the superior intelligence, the ability to succeed in college or in the teaching profession, or to learn that they were not attractive to others and were not liked.

Every day, people are learning these facts. Some are able to accept them; others are not. What is relevant at this point is that the regard one has of one's self, or the "picture" one has of one's self, or the "self-concept," is on a level of importance with one's body. And a threat to the first as, for example, "You are not college material," can be as great a blow as a threat to the second, for example, "You have diabetes." The self is "body-plus," body plus all those aspects of the world which the individual perceives "as definite and fairly stable characteristics of himself."[4] Self includes his identity with a particular family, with a girl or boy friend, with a professional group, and a threat to his continued affiliation with these is a threat to self, against which he must set up defenses. These, as much as a physical body, are the attributes of the self which he must maintain and enhance. Disabled veterans, unable to accept themselves in their new status, refuse to return to their families; the young man, rejected by the object of his affection and unable to accept himself in this status, leaves town; the young pitcher in the minor leagues, new to professional baseball, unable to accept himself in the status of a losing pitcher after losing one game and being taken out of the second, goes from ball park to railroad station where he buys a ticket for a destination far removed from his team's itinerary.

While survival of the physical body is important, there are many persons who will knowingly endanger it in an attempt to achieve certain personal goals, such as wealth and educational attainment, in order to enhance the other aspects of self. For them there does not seem to be a choice they could rationally consider between desirable bodily care and excessively high levels of aspiration. For example, a man sees himself as a successful professional man, and has the need to be one. If the attainment of that status threatens to impair his physical condition, he will lower his goal only if he can so reorganize his self-picture that being another kind of worker will maintain and enhance this newly organized self.

Jack, a veteran, twenty-four years old, now a college sophomore in an engineering curriculum, was referred to the

[4] Donald Snygg and Arthur W. Combs, *Individual Behavior: A New Frame of Reference for Psychology,* New York: Harper and Bros., 1949; p. 112.

counselor by the college physician. Jack had gone to the health center because of his fatigue. The physician found no organic ailment. He asked Jack how much sleep he had been getting, and Jack said, an average of five hours a night. No wonder he was tired! He asked the physician for a prescription to reduce the fatigue, explaining that it would be impossible to get more sleep.

During several counseling interviews, the following facts emerged. Jack came from an underprivileged home. He had always been interested in books, but he had known when he entered high school that he would have to work part-time and that he would be fortunate if he could finish high school, and that he would have little chance to go to college.

While in the Army, he developed a great respect and admiration for several engineer officers. Being an engineer became to him synonymous with being important and successful. When he learned of the G I Bill of Rights, he decided that he would go to college and become an engineer. Life at college was one endless grind. Admiring his persistence, but pitying him for his inaptitude, instructors advised him to change his course. While the evidence of his lack of qualification was abundant, he could not accept it, for it was contrary to his needs for self-enhancement. During one interview he shouted, "I'll go on until I drop. I've *got* to be an engineer." The status of engineer was more important to him than the condition of his body.

After a series of interviews Jack decided that he would transfer to another program of study. He had found it possible now to maintain and enhance himself without being an engineer.

One often hears the remark: "I did it (or did not do it) because otherwise I wouldn't be able to live with myself." People find one means or another to make it possible to live with themselves. On the one hand, they alter the self-picture so that it is more in accord with reality. For example, the college freshman whose goal is medicine, finally accepts the fact that he cannot achieve this goal and is prepared to "live with himself" as an X-ray technician. On the other hand, they succeed in living with themselves by maintaining the self-picture by such devices as achievement, overachievement, rationalization, daydreaming, delusioning, alcoholism. If our theory is valid, those who can do neither, that is, neither maintain the self-concept nor change it, commit suicide.

From birth to death all the specific needs of the individual are embraced by the maintenance and enhancement of self. The infant's need to suckle and to be held, to be clothed and sheltered are part of this broader need. So, too, are the child's need to feel loved by his parents and accepted by his peers, the adolescent's need to gain freedom from the family and to feel attractive to the opposite sex, the adult's need for status in an occupation and in a family. All are encompassed by the over-all need to feel that this "I" survives and is well regarded, that "it belongs," is accepted, recognized, and admired. They are all part of this need of mine that the picture of myself that I accept, the one that now makes life worth living, is accepted by others, is maintained and even enhanced; that I am thought of not only as a teacher (or pitcher, dancer, speaker, lover, wife, father), but as a good one at that.

The emphasis on "self" possibly suggests that this interpretation of human behavior (based on our two assumptions) excludes altruism, social cooperation, international peace. This is not so. In his drive toward maturity and the satisfaction of the need for maintenance and enhancement of self, the individual adopts or internalizes the values of his society, particularly of the subcultures and the social institutions which influence him. If he learns that prestige, status, respect, admiration, "belonging" (as well as the satisfaction of physiological drives) comes from cooperation and public service, then these will be characteristic of the skills he will acquire in his drive toward growth, health, and maturity. Then the picture-of-self with which he will live will be of a person with these characteristics.

Recapitulation. The counselor can work effectively only when he understands the dynamics of behavior of his clients. Despite differences among people in their characteristics of personality and in their behavior, they are all moved by the same basic force, the need to maintain and enhance the self. This need is satisfied by a drive toward life, growth, health, and maturity. At birth, the drive is characterized by reflex acts that promote survival and development, and subsequently by learned patterns of behavior as well as by the simpler reflexes.

The Evolution of Self

We turn now to the development of self. We note how an individual living in one social circle, under one set of social pressures becomes an adequate or "well-adjusted" self, capable of dealing with life's problems, whereas another individual in another social circle, under different social pressures becomes an inadequate or "maladjusted" self, incapable of dealing with his problems. As health counselors most of our efforts are devoted to the second individual to aid him in achieving the adequacy that will permit him to solve his problems.

Just as the notion that some children are born "bad" has been discarded, so has been the equally outdated one that some are born maladjusted. Even the assertion that some are born with a predisposition to emotional disturbance or to personality disintegration has no basis in fact. Surely, the child born with abnormality in structure, such as lack of one hand, or in facial appearance, such as extreme ugliness of feature, is greatly handicapped in his efforts at need-satisfaction. This is so not because of the predisposition within himself, but rather because of the manner in which people react to him. Stated differently, he regards himself as an undesirable, unacceptable person because he has seen himself so mirrored, so pictured in the attitudes and behavior of his family, his playmates and neighbors. He learned that he was not acceptable when he noticed children stare at a stump where a hand should have been, when he sensed that adults avoided touching it or heard them whisper, "What a pity!" People in his world taught him to see himself as an undesirable person and led him to withdraw into a hermit's world where his self would not be threatened by these perceptions, but a world which would not satisfy his needs. Development of his inadequate self was not predestined by his structural deficiency; it was the result of the behavior of others and of the lessons he learned from them.

So it is with all persons. The kind of self one develops and its adequacy for need-satisfaction are a product of perceptions and learning. The individual interacts with his society. He learns about himself from others. The new learning leads to changes in behavior. The changed behavior produces different responses from persons in his environment, which, in turn, lead to new learning, changed behavior, different responses, and other changes.

Comparison of adequate and inadequate selves. Some persons can achieve accurate perception of their self and their world, and others cannot. Thus, some people have a self-picture that corresponds in large measure to the picture that more objective observers have of them; others have a self-picture, however, that is at sharp variance with the perceptions of observers. To some persons, a change in their circumstances, for better or for worse, is clearly perceived as such and in one way or another is integrated in their lives. To others, a change in circumstances becomes a distorted perception; it is misshapen, magnified, or dwarfed. The perceptions of some people are in accord with reality, and since behavior is based on perceptions of self and world, their behavior is based on adequate data, and is adequate. The perceptions of other people are as accurate as those one gets when looking into the distorted, curved mirrors at an amusement park, and the behavior that stems from such inadequate data is itself inadequate. Let us further examine this concept of adequacy as it is illustrated in cases.

One man clearly perceives at forty-five that he is aging, that aging is a normal, irrevocable, acceptable phenomenon, and adapts his behavior to it by such safeguards of his health as participation in a less active competitive sport, such as golf. Another man, who perceives aging as unattractive and devoid of satisfaction and thus as a threat to maintenance and enhancement of self, declares "You're as old as you feel," and at forty-five plays basketball and dates twenty-year-old girls.

One man clearly perceives that he is different from the normal in the absence of a limb, that he is stared on and pitied by strangers. He does not like what he sees, but he sees clearly, and he adapts his behavior by proceeding to seek a job, a wife, and a family that can help him satisfy his needs for self-enhancement. Another man distortedly views the same set of circumstances: he sees himself as utterly useless, unattractive and rejected. He must learn to maintain and enhance his self by other means, such as daydreaming, overemphasis of some activity in which he is skillful, or self-aggrandizement even by antisocial behavior. He regards himself as a burden and interprets any attempts to assist him as pity for his deformed condition. These distorted perceptions are further reinforced by the refusal of an employer to hire him, by the unsolicited offers of strangers to help him cross the street, or by the momentary hesitation of a girl at his invitation to dance.[5]

One college coed, age nineteen, five feet ten inches in

[5] Those who attempt to motivate amputees and other physically disabled persons by emphasizing their normality to the complete disregard of their very real physical shortcomings and society's reaction to them do these people an injustice. Their self-pictures are not in accord with reality. Yet, on the basis of the distorted perceptions, they thrust themselves on to an employer for jobs for which they are not qualified, and they seek the same acceptance in social relationships they had previously known. The rejection they receive from the employer, and the curious stare and hesitant reaction from strangers and even from friends and relatives may drive them to solitude as an escape.

height, clearly perceives herself as being decidedly taller than the average girl, and taller even than the average male on the campus. She recognizes certain disadvantages as, for example, when she shops for clothing, but she is more often aware of the advantages in "standing out from the crowd," as when she is elected a class officer. She shows her pride and satisfaction in her posture and social poise.[6] Another coed of the same age and same height has since early adolescence regarded this characteristic as a curse on her. Having heard relatives and neighbors predict a variety of unwelcome consequences ("Won't she ever stop growing?" "How will she find a fellow tall enough for her?"), she has learned to regard her height as something unlovely and unacceptable, something that is to be avoided. Thus, she stands hunched and round-shouldered, distorting her posture in order not to stand out from the crowd.

One high-school junior accurately perceives that his complexion is badly marred by acne eruptions, but he sees this in perspective with his many positive qualities. Consequently, while seeking medical attention to improve his complexion, he continues relatively unimpaired the social relationships necessary for need-satisfaction of the adolescent. Another high-school junior with the same condition views it out of focus. As if he had been looking into our wavy amusement park mirror which magnified the eruptions a hundredfold, he has been overwhelmed, seeing its significance entirely out of proportion to reality. He sits in classes with other people, but is not part of a group. He does not "belong," and his attitudes toward his self and the type of behavior they produce are inadequate for need-satisfaction.

As we examine the differentiating characteristic of the pairs of persons described, we find that one in each pair was able to adapt to new circumstances in his or her life: growing old, losing a limb, growing exceedingly tall, and developing poor

[6] This wholesome acceptance of height is demonstrated in the Tall Girls' Clubs.

complexion. Each of these persons perceived a new phenomenon in life, recognized it as reality, and made whatever changes were necessary in his mode of living in order to adjust to the new fact. These persons need not have liked what they perceived; surely the amputee did not welcome the change, but they accepted what they recognized as reality and they reorganized their self-pictures and their behavior in order to continue to be able to satisfy their needs in efficient and practical ways. Each continued about his business of being part of a group and enjoying the respect of his peers.

This was not true of the opposite member of each pair. They, too, reacted to a set of new physical stimuli, the same stimuli that acted on the others. Although the stimuli were the same, the perceptions were different. To these poorly adjusted individuals, the meanings attached to the stimuli were qualitatively different from those of their opposites. Different meaning made for different perception; different perception suggested different behavior. Meanings given to stimuli represent a personal accretion to the realities of the world. To each individual, what is real is not the stimulus alone as it exists in the external world; reality is the stimulus and personal accretion, the combination of which make for a perception. The personal accretion lends the stimulus a connotation to the perceiver, adding some further meaning to the precise one it possesses in definition made by a variety of observers.

The accretions to the stimuli of our four adequate persons did not distort reality. What was real for them was sufficiently in accord with the external world so that their actions were neither bizarre nor fruitless. For example, our forty-five year old man, noting his fatigue after a strenuous set of tennis doubles, recalls a statement of his father's made many years earlier that as one matures one finds so many more satisfactions in life. For him, aging is associated with gain as well as loss. His outlook on it does not interfere with his efforts at need-satisfaction. Not so with his opposite. This forty-five year old man who perceives aging as a termination of satisfying living, as a threat to his self, cannot halt the ravages of age by playing basketball. In fact, he may invite them earlier. So long as satisfaction is linked to youthfulness, he is doomed to decreasing satisfactions in life. The meaning he has learned to give to aging *does* get in *his* way. It prevents efficiency in his attempt to satisfy his needs.

One of our tall coeds glories in her height which she has converted into an asset through poise and good posture. Not so the other, who, perceiving her height as a threat to attractive femininity, avoids the spotlight in school and nonschool social activity, thus diminishing the opportunity to develop social skills. The meaning she has given to her height has now made her unskilled in social behavior and unattractive. Thus, the meaning she has learned to associate with height has given a threatening cast to her perception and has made need-satisfaction difficult to achieve.

In our four maladjusted individuals, the real cause of maladjustment was not the physical or health condition, for the other member of the pair was able to adjust. The manner in which each of them regarded his new circumstances caused the maladjustment. It was not aging, acne, height, or amputation that made life difficult and created problems that brought four people to a specialist. It was the meaning given to aging, acne, height, and amputation that brought them there; just as different meanings, and thus different behavior, made it necessary for the other member of the four pairs to seek aid.

Our four maladjusted people are not stupid, ignorant, or uncooperative, though they create unhappiness for themselves and for others. Their problems can no more be corrected by confinement, harsh discipline, or logical reasoning than that of a five-year-old lad in a temper tantrum. Their perceptions, which have made life difficult for them, are a product of meanings attached to the stimuli. For us who seek to help these people, the task is to aid them in changing these meanings. We provide the sincerity of interest and the professional skill that will enable our four people to perceive aging, amputation, height, and acne in less threatening terms. In the permissive atmosphere of the counseling interview, threat is removed and the four clients have the opportunity to bring their perceptions into greater harmony with objective reality.

Questions

1. What enables you to maintain and enhance your self?
2. To what extent is (or was) college attendance related to your self-enhancement?
3. In what ways has the drive for health, growth and maturity been reflected in your own life?
4. Have any of your attitudes, as for example toward people, behavior, work, play, religion, politics, or sex, ever been revised? If so, what brought about this revision?

Bibliography

Arbuckle, Dugald S., *Teacher Counseling,* Cambridge: Addison-Wesley, 1950, chapters 2 and 3.

Bingham, Walter V. D., and Bruce V. Moore, *How to Interview,* New York: Harper and Bros., 1941, chapter 1.

Hahn, Milton E., and Malcolm S. MacLean, *General Clinical Counseling,* New York: McGraw-Hill, 1950, chapter 2.

Hamrin, Shirley A., and Blanche B. Paulson, *Counseling Adolescents,* Chicago: Science Research Associates, 1950, chapters 3 and 4.

Rogers, Carl R., *Counseling and Psychotherapy,* New York: Houghton Mifflin Co., 1942, parts I and II.

Rogers, Carl R., *Client-Centered Therapy,* New York: Houghton Mifflin Co., 1951, chapter I.

Snygg, Donald, and Arthur W. Combs, *Individual Behavior, A New Frame of Reference for Psychology,* New York: Harper and Bros., 1949. An interpretation of human behavior that is meaningful even to those untrained in psychology.

Strang, Ruth, *Counseling Technics in College and Secondary*

School, New York: Harper and Bros., 1949. See chapter 6 for discussion of the varied counseling orientations.

Williamson, E. G., *Counseling Adolescents,* New York: McGraw-Hill, 1950. A counseling orientation diametrically opposed to ours.

Chapter IV

THE DESIRABLE QUALITIES OF THE HEALTH COUNSELOR

The role of the counselor's personality is as important in the study of counseling as it is in the counseling relationship itself. The desirable characteristics are discussed at this time because they grow out of the philosophy of counseling and they, in turn, determine the dynamics and techniques described in subsequent chapters. For example, a basic principle already discussed is that each individual has the capacity to reorganize his concepts of self and his world. This requires a counselor whose personality permits him to respect the right of the individual to make his own decisions and who has learned the skills of creating the atmosphere in which this goal can be achieved.

Whether his client is an amputee, an arrested tuberculosis case, a high-school boy with rheumatic heart, an unmarried mother, or a woman at menopause, the counselor sets himself the task of helping the client recognize and accept[1] the realities of his self and his world. He seeks to accomplish this by creating a special type of environment that encourages a mature approach to life. Part of that environment is the counselor himself. In order that the counselor can create the psy-

[1] "Acceptance" by the client does not imply resignation; it is a recognition of reality that leads him to positive action.

chological climate that promotes change, he must have certain attitudes toward people and himself and in addition certain skills and knowledge. These attitudes are treated separately on the following pages, but they are not separate and distinct. Attitudes toward one's self and others are interrelated, and acceptance of one's self appears to be accompanied by acceptance of others.[2]

Attitudes Toward People

One of the basic ingredients in job satisfaction is a strong liking for the materials with which one works. The "materials" of the counselor are people. The counselor who dislikes people cannot serve them well professionally and will very likely be an unhappy worker. A strong liking for people is an essential quality of the counselor.

He must like them simply because they are people and not because he achieves personal satisfaction from using or manipulating them. It is conceivable that a person who has the title of counselor can dislike people, yet gain satisfaction from his job, because it enables him to express his hostility for them, to exploit and abuse them.

The concept of liking as it is used here refers to the outward expression of an attitude that people are of supreme worth. This kind of liking leads to positive feelings and is a "moving out toward people" that is reflected even in the highly attentive posture and expression of the counselor as he listens to and shares the expressed feelings of the client. It is reflected in the behavior of the counselor who cannot sit stiff-necked behind an executive desk and issue pontifical prescriptions of behavior to a client.

The kind of person who cannot be a counselor is characterized by the final lines from an excerpt from *The Lonesome Train, A Musical Legend.*[3] These musical records, which

[2] Elizabeth T. Sheerer, "The Relationship between Acceptance of Self and of Others," *Journal of Consulting Psychology,* 13, 169-175 (1949).

[3] Music by Earl Robinson, words by Millard Lampell, directed by Norman Corwin, Decca Album No. DA-375, 1944.

trace the journey of Lincoln's body from Washington, D. C., to Springfield, Illinois, seek to express the very essence of that which was Lincoln. The narrator tells of the great masses of people who mourned at his bier. But there were exceptions. There were those who profited because Lincoln was dead, and they celebrated.

> Yes, there were those who cheered:
> The Copperheads;
> a New York politician who didn't like Lincoln;
> an Ohio businessman who didn't like Negroes;
> a Chicago newspaper editor who didn't like people.

The potential health counselor can check for himself if his liking and respect for people are sufficiently broad in scope to permit him to serve his clients. In examining the following list he can judge whether he is truly interested in the adjustment problems of the diverse people who make up the clientele of the counselor. He can answer questions like the following: Can I shake the hand of this person and warmly welcome him? Am I really interested in helping him deal with his problem? Can I truly accept him as he is and make him comfortable and trusting enough to come to grips with his problem? Place a check mark next to each group for which your answer to the last question is "no."

White
Negro
Oriental

Catholic
Jew
Protestant
Quaker
Christian Scientist
Seventh Day Adventist
Atheist
English

Scandinavian
French
Italian
American
Russian
Turkish
Chinese
American Indian
Asiatic Indian
Polish
Irish
Syrian

Armenian
Mexican
Puerto Rican
German
Spanish

Amputee
Cerebral palsy child

Infantile paralysis patient
Acne case
Unmarried mother
Sexually promiscuous high school junior
Homosexual student
Arrested tuberculosis case
Blind person

QUESTIONS

1. How limited would your clientele be?
2. Could you serve all the students in the public school in which you now work, or would like to work, or in the schools you have attended?

A half dozen adults have come to visit in a home in which the five year old son is playing on the floor with toy cars and trucks. Each of the adults is introduced to Johnny and each attempts to attract his interest, but only one succeeds. Why does he succeed? Let us examine the methods that several of these adults used, reading the lines aloud as we would expect them to be spoken. Decide for yourself the feelings that each of these adults evokes in Johnny. Our version of his reactions appears at the end of this chapter.

The first adult says: "What a nice little man you are, playing so quietly and not bothering anyone!"

The second adult says: "And what are *you* going to be when you grow up, Mr. Johnny, a truck driver?" He laughs as he says this and turns to the other adults for reaction to his joke.

The third one remarks: "Say, that's not the way the trucks go on the road. You'll have them all in a collision. Now let me show you how to do it."

The fourth one loudly says: "What a big boy. Come on,

put up your mitts and let's go a few rounds," as he lightly taps the child's face.

The fifth one says quietly: "Hello, Johnny. May I sit down and play with you?"

The first four adults may like children but they do not respect them as individuals. They feel that children are tiny persons, easy to exploit for one's own purposes and not deserving of the respect that these adults themselves would demand of others. To the fifth adult, Johnny is a human, as worthy of respect as the head of a government, the prelate of a church, or the distinguished member of a high-prestige profession, such as medicine.

This illustration has its counterpart in attitudes of high school and college students toward faculty members. "He's different," they will say about the teacher who treats his students with a dignity sometimes reserved only for supervisors. Such a teacher does not regard the students as necessary evils who interfere with research, writing, and other pursuits.

Respect for people means respect for *all* people, regardless of age, sex, race, religion, political creed, income, family status, education, achievement, health, physical appearance, physical or mental limitations. This assertion does not stem from a political creed. It is not even made in order to insure that the counselor is prepared to serve all types of persons, for there is frequently an opportunity to refer a client with whom one cannot work effectively to another counselor. The assertion is made because respect for people can have no limits without altering the quality of the relationship. To say, "I respect the integrity of all individuals except those of a particular group, such as unmarried mothers," is comparable to saying there are humans who do not deserve respect, and it implies that the speaker entertains the right to add others to a subhuman status. Such a statement also implies that the person has a need to place others in an inferior position.

Like Johnny, clients are quick to sense the attitudes of the counselor to them. If they do not perceive a genuine warmth and interest and an essential dignity, they cannot develop a profitable counseling relationship. When the counselor accepts a client with a dignity reserved for humans, he enables the client to develop a sense of worthiness and respect for himself.

The importance of this respect in the reorganization of an individual's outlook and behavior is indicated in a bit of character delineation from Act V of Shaw's *Pygmalion.* Liza Doolittle, a flower girl with cockney dialect, goes to the home of Professor Henry Higgins for speech instruction. She hopes correct speech will help her rise from her present position to that of a lady in a flower shop. Colonel Pickering, a friend of Higgins, bets the professor that he cannot transform Liza into a lady before the date of the ambassador's garden party. During the subsequent weeks Liza is transformed into a beautiful, charming lady and Higgins wins the bet. In the same period Liza falls in love with him, and he, though unaware of it, with her.

After the party, Liza and Higgins become involved in a bitter argument. Higgins' scientific detachment from the subject of his experiment and his satisfaction at its termination revive and reinforce Liza's feelings of inferior position and infuriate her. She leaves the house. Higgins and Pickering engage in a vigorous search. They find her unexpectedly at the home of Higgins' mother.

> *Higgins:* You let her alone, mother. Let her speak for herself. You will jolly soon see whether she has an idea that I havnt put into her head or a word that I havnt put into her mouth. I tell you I have created this thing out of the squashed cabbage leaves of Covent Garden; and now she pretends to play the fine lady with me.
>
> *Mrs. Higgins* (placidly): Yes, dear; but you'll sit down, wont you?
>
> Higgins sits down again, savagely.

Liza (to Pickering, taking no apparent notice of Higgins, and working away deftly [with her needlework]): Will you drop me altogether now that the experiment is over, Colonel Pickering?

Pickering: Oh dont. You mustnt think of it as an experiment. It shocks me, somehow.

Liza: Oh, I'm only a squashed cabbage leaf—

Pickering (impulsively): No.

Liza (continuing quietly)—but I owe so much to you that I should be very unhappy if you forgot me.

Pickering: It's very kind of you to say so, Miss Doolittle.

Liza: It's not because you paid for my dresses. I know you are generous to everybody with money. But it was from you that I learnt really nice manners; and that is what makes one a lady, isnt it? You see it was so very difficult for me with the example of Professor Higgins always before me. I was brought up to be just like him, unable to control myself, and using bad language on the slightest provocation. And I should never have known that ladies and gentlemen didnt behave like that if you hadnt been there.

Higgins: Well!!

Pickering: Oh, thats only his way, you know He doesnt mean it.

Liza: Oh, *I* didnt mean it either, when I was a flower girl. It was only my way. But you see I did it; and thats what makes the difference after all.

Pickering: No doubt. Still, he taught you to speak; and I couldnt have done that, you know.

Liza (trivially): Of course: that is his profession.

Higgins: Damnation!

Liza (continuing): It was just like learning to dance in the fashionable way: there was nothing more than that in it. But do you know what began my real education?

Pickering: What?

Liza (stopping her work for a moment): Your calling me Miss Doolittle that day when I first came to Wimpole Street. That was the beginning of self-respect for me. (She resumes her stitching.) And there were a hundred little things you never noticed, because they came naturally to you. Things about standing up and taking off your hat and opening doors—

Pickering: Oh, that was nothing.

Liza: Yes: things that shewed you thought and felt about me as if I were something better than a scullery-maid; though of course I know you would have been just the same to a scullery-maid if she had been let into the drawing room. You never took off your boots in the dining room when I was there.

Pickering: You mustnt mind that. Higgins takes off his boots all over the place.

Liza: I know. I am not blaming him. It is his way, isnt it? But it made such a difference to me that you didnt do it. You see, really and truly, apart from the things anyone can pick up (the dressing and the proper way of speaking, and so on), the difference between a lady and a flower girl is not how she behaves, but how she's treated. I shall always be a flower girl to Professor Higgins, because he always treats me as a flower girl, and always will; but I know I can be a lady to you, because you always treat me as a lady, and always will.[4]

When this healthy respect for people is translated into the counselor-client relation during an interview, the counselor does not assume that he knows the course the interview must take or the experiences or problems of the client which are most important for discussion. He does not take on himself the inviolable right of each individual to make decisions concerning his own behavior.

Acceptance of people's feelings is inseparable from respect. The counselor who creates the permissive atmosphere in which clients feel free to express themselves will hear them talk of their fears, hatreds, anxieties, and inadequacies. He will hear descriptions of socially disapproved behavior, such

[4] Bernard Shaw, *Selected Plays with Prefaces,* New York: Dodd Mead and Company, 1948, p. 269 and 270. Copyright by George Bernard Shaw. Reprinted by permission of the Public Trustee and the Society of Authors.

as sexual perversion, delinquency, deep parental hatred, "sacrilegious" feelings, and extreme political views. These he must be able to accept if he is to serve his clients.

Acceptance of the attitudes, feelings, and behavior of people as used in connection with counseling does not involve any value except the inherent respect for people. The counselor neither approves nor disapproves of any of the following client statements. He only accepts them as the valid feelings of the client at the moment they are expressed:

> You teachers are all the same—you all think I'm a bad girl.
>
> My old man can go straight to the devil as far as I'm concerned. He's never lifted a finger to make me happy.
>
> My wife!—all she ever wanted of me was money. Now that I want to leave her she talks of love.
>
> What kind of a God would make me lose my arm?
>
> Tuberculosis? Me? (with a dazed expression) I can't believe it . . . I don't want to live if it's true.

The client-centered counselor neither approves nor disapproves of these feelings. Liking and respecting his client as a human being, he as much as says:

> I understand your feelings; I don't approve or disapprove of them, but I accept them and trust that you will feel free to continue to express—perhaps for the first time in your life—these feelings that would not be acceptable elsewhere.
>
> Tell me, if you like, that you are frightened to go to the dentist, and I will not laugh at you or even tell you that, of course, the dentist will not injure you. Tell me that you dislike the changes in your body, that you are ashamed of your dreams, that you masturbate and hate yourself for it; that life means very little if you cannot see, or walk, or hear; tell me these things and I will accept them and respect you; and I will allow you to come to see that you, too, can

accept these feelings, and accept and respect yourself, that you can maintain and enhance this self of yours.

The counselor's attitude is akin to that of Voltaire's classic statement about philosophical differences, "I disapprove of what you say, but I will defend to the death your right to say it." The counselor paraphrases this by thinking:

> I may or may not agree with your feelings, but it is my professional responsibility to create the atmosphere in which you can say it freely without fear of criticism, reprisal, approval, or disapproval; and whatever you say will meet with my acceptance. You may or may not be the kind of person whom I'd like as a relative, friend, or colleague, but you are human, and whatever there is about you that is unsavory to me was produced by your inheritance or environment operating in this society. I understand this and accept it.

Attitudes Toward Self

An important characteristic of the counselor is an understanding of himself and the effect of his self on others. This can be seen most clearly when considering the external attributes of the counselor.

The physically attractive female counselor induces more than just a counselor-client relationship with a male client during the early stages of the interview. To deny this is to deny reality. The counselor can be most effective when she is aware of her sexual attraction, understands it, accepts it, and then provides the atmosphere in which the client can recognize that this feeling of his, like all others, is accepted and respected. He discovers the uniqueness of this relationship in which his values are neither rejected nor even challenged by the counselor. This could be achieved, however, only when the counselor can understand and can handle the effect of herself on the client.

The counselor in the school or college finds that the client's initial reaction to him is similar to the client's reaction to a teacher or administrator. The student knows that the teacher is a person who judges his work and grades him, and who sometimes criticizes him for not doing his assignment or for not knowing the lesson. Coming to a counselor for the first time, the student regards him as an authoritarian person. If the client is guarded in his remarks, hesitant and fearful to express feelings that might be socially disapproved, the counselor understands the effect of his self as a school official on the client. He seeks to alter the meaning he has for the student by his behavior, his genuine respect for and acceptance of him.

Failure to understand this and to deal with it will leave the counselor a much less effective person than otherwise. It will also delimit his ability to evaluate his interviews, for lack of progress and failure are sometimes the result of the counselor's lack of sensitivity to his effect on the client.

Some counselors are outgoing persons, skilled at first introductions; others are more reserved, more serious. No one type of personality has been found characteristic of counselor success. However, the counselor needs to know that the client is going to be affected by his personality. The young counselor, insecure in his first experience, possibly threatened by client statements which he feels unequipped to handle as effectively as he would like to, can nevertheless achieve success if he understands the impact of his reactions on the client and learns how to deal with it.

The counselor must know himself well enough to identify his limitations. He must be able to recognize when he can be of no further service to a client, and when the client should be referred to a more skilled or more specialized professional worker. He must also know when the client can benefit from supplementary service from another worker. The person who regards referral to another person as a reflection on himself is too immature to serve as counselor. The health counselor must work with other specialists in human relations, including other professional counselors, teachers, physicians, psychologists, coaches, clergymen, and social workers.

Most health counselors must work as part of a team. It is questionable that a counselor in the school can serve students effectively without cooperative arrangements with the school physician, nurse, educational and vocational counselor, and especially with the teachers. The following case illustrates this team work.

> Miss Smith, tenth-grade home room teacher, noticed that Mary seemed to have no friends and to be unhealthily quiet and asocial. Miss Smith made a special effort to gain Mary's confidence. One day, after a discussion that Miss Smith had initiated on the health services in the school, Mary asked if she would talk with her. Miss Smith suggested they talk after school.
>
> During the first interview, Mary indicated that she hated being a girl, that she did not really understand what happened each month to make her feel so upset. Miss Smith did not tell Mary to be proud that she was a girl, nor did she take over the interview and commence to lecture Mary on the facts of life. Yes, she knew that the facts were important and that Mary should become familiar with them, but she was aware that until Mary's negative feelings about being a girl and about menstruating were dealt with, the facts would be of little value.
>
> Miss Smith gave Mary the opportunity to express these feelings, and she, as counselor, accepted them and encouraged her to talk. At the end of a half hour Miss Smith asked Mary if she would like to talk with her like this again. Mary said, "Yes." Miss Smith set aside half an hour each week. During the third week Mary spoke of excessive pain during menstruation. Miss Smith asked if she would like a physical examination to see if the pain could be reduced. When Mary requested this, Miss Smith referred her to the nurse. Mary asked also if the nurse could explain the bodily processes to her.

> Miss Smith spoke with the nurse prior to Mary's visit to the health office. As Mary began to show a desire to socialize more, Miss Smith also spoke with her other teachers to enlist their aid in helping Mary enter into activities and achieve some early success and satisfactions. During this whole period, Miss Smith was in touch with the school's full-time counselor. At the conclusion of the counseling, she prepared a brief report for Mary's cumulative record so that those who would work with Mary in the future could better understand her; that any deficiencies in her grades during the period of unhappiness or the period of change could be explained; and that previous descriptions of her asocial behavior should not remain unexplained on her record, handicapping her unfairly by giving the reader an inaccurate picture of the girl.

The same understanding of self that is important in the counseling relationship is also important in the teamwork of health counselor with other members of faculty and staff. A healthy respect for each person's attitudes and his acceptance as an equal are far more satisfactory than the unfortunately prevalent attitude that the counselor is an administrator who uses the faculty to achieve the goals that *he* sees as important by the methods that *he* regards as desirable.

Effective counseling in a school, in a hospital, in a school of nursing, in a community agency is possible only if the various members of the faculty and staff are conscious of the need for counseling and are aware of their roles in the program. To accomplish this, the counselor who is responsible, e.g., for the school's guidance program plans activities that will permit the faculty to participate fully and genuinely in the activation and development of the counseling program. This demands of the counselor a personality that will not regard as a threat the growing participation of others in his field of specialization. The health counselor has a more limited range of activity, but the effectiveness of his work is no less dependent on an understanding, cooperative relationship with the faculty.

The counseling relationship described here is a unique one. While it has many of the characteristics of other professional relations, there are distinct differences. The counselor does not examine the client, diagnose the problem, and prescribe a course of action as a cure. He does not urge the client to seek solace in his religion or to exchange his values for those of his church. He does not claim to be able to teach the client the correct way to live. His function is different and unique: to aid the client to discover that way of life which the client finds to be best for him, no matter at what variance that may be with the counselor's own way of life. The amputee has the right to decide that it is difficult for him to expose his "being different" to strangers, and that he prefers to direct his educational and vocational planning toward a career that does not involve public contact; or to decide that he enjoys the attention and advantages that his "being different" elicits, and that he prefers to plan for a public contact job. The client's decision may be contrary to what the counselor believes he would have made in the same situation, but the counselor knows that his decision would be right for himself and that the client's decision is right for the client.

Desirable Skills and Knowledge

The warm accepting relationship is the basis of effective counseling. Without this, there can be no counseling. The essentiality of this may be emphasized by the fact that all counseling orientations claim this as a basic principle.

A significant study by Fiedler[5] has given us the concept of the "Ideal Counseling Relationship." The keystone of this relationship is the counselor's ability to participate completely in the client's communication. To state it differently, the counselor knows what the client is trying to convey to

[5] Fred E. Fiedler, "The Concept of the Ideal Therapeutic Relationship," *Journal of Consulting Psychology,* 14, 239-245 (1950).

him, and the client is aware that the counselor knows. A second and equally significant investigation by Fiedler[6] compared the counselor-client relationship of an experienced and of an inexperienced counselor from each of three different major schools of counseling. He found that experts created a relationship closer to the ideal than nonexperts; he also found that experts, regardless of the school of counseling, created a relationship more like other experts than like the nonexperts from their own school of counseling. Finally, "the most important dimension (of those measured) which differentiates experts from nonexperts is related to the therapist's ability to understand, to communicate with, and to maintain rapport with the (client)." [7]

The most essential skill of the counselor is his ability to recognize the feelings of his client and to reflect them. The counselor must be able to experience the feelings of another person. As the client verbalizes his attitudes toward himself, his handicaps, his ailments, and toward other people, the counselor seeks to understand the client and identify the feeling in the client's words, gestures, and facial expressions. Since self-understanding by the client is the goal in counseling, the counselor seeks to facilitate this by understanding his client's feelings. These are sometimes veiled by ambiguity of expression that the client uses in self-protection, in fear that this stranger will reject him for his feelings. These feelings are then highlighted through statements that clarify them. To see these skills in action, note the response of the counselor to the following client statements:

> *Twenty year old college sophomore:* So I have a bad heart! Who cares! I'm going to go on the way I am and enjoy life while I live instead of vegetating many years.

[6] Fred E. Fiedler, "A Comparison of Therapeutic Relationships in Psychoanalytic, Nondirective and Adlerian Therapy," *Journal of Consulting Psychology*, 14, 436-445 (1950).
[7] *Ibid.*, p. 444.

Counselor: Life isn't worth living for you unless you go on the same way.

High school sophomore girl (who has resisted attending health class): I don't really know what it is I don't like about it. The teacher's all right, but the things she talks about! And the way the girls talk! Sometimes it makes me feel—well, just dirty.

Counselor: You get upset and feel there is something wrong in this talk about the body.

The counselor has crystallized the feeling embedded in the client's words and gestures. This process, explained in greater detail in subsequent chapters, and the skills required for it are essential to counseling that regards the client's feelings as the chief focus.

The health counselor should be familiar with the general symptoms of deviation from good physical and emotional health. He should understand the medical terminology on the health record used in his institution and recognize its import to the educational, vocational, and social activities of the client.

The health counselor is dependent on the other professional workers in his organization and on other professional resources in the community. His knowledge of services such as the following can make the difference between success and failure in a counseling case: special placement service for the handicapped; financial aid in securing dentures; organized social activities for adolescents and the aged; free or low-cost psychiatric service.

Other valuable skills are as follows:

(1) Leadership of case conference discussions. The health counselor occasionally finds it profitable and has the time to arrange for a meeting of the teachers or institutional staff members who have contact with the client. The purposes of the meeting are to familiarize them with the problem, to share information about the student, to develop a well-integrated team in working with him, and to contribute to the

coordination of the school's counseling program. Such conferences tend to sensitize the concerned staff members to the needs of the client.

(2) The anecdotal report, cumulative record, autobiography, adjustment inventory, case study. While the stress in this book is on the interview as the chief instrument in counseling, these tools and techniques are useful in helping locate those students—there are a great many of them—who do not know of the counseling service and who welcome the counselor's aid when they learn it is available. These tools are particularly useful with unmotivated students who are afraid of counseling and do not make themselves known, or who are not living efficiently yet are not sufficiently motivated to seek help. These are discussed more fully in Chapter VII.

(3) Group discussion leadership. Economy of time demands much health counseling to be performed with groups of students. Group discussions under the leadership of a skilled person can serve the remedial purposes of counseling as well as the preventive purposes of health education. In addition, group discussion, with the same permissive atmosphere as in individual counseling, has therapeutic value. It can help bring about some of the changes in a person's outlook and behavior that are the goal of counseling. The physically handicapped child finds that he is not alone in the feelings of inadequacy. The reserved individual has an opportunity to develop social skills. The principles of counseling with the individual are in most respects transferable to the group situation.

In the case described on page 52, Johnny's feelings toward each of the five adults were:

> *To the first:* I wish he wouldn't bother me.
>
> *To the second:* He's trying to be funny.
>
> *To the third:* I don't like him. He's breaking up my game. He thinks he knows it all.
>
> *To the fourth* (as he moves away): I don't like that bad man.
>
> *To the fifth* (as he makes room for this adult): I like him.

Questions

1. For which of your own qualities do you have the greatest respect? For which, the least respect?
2. What are the qualities in others that you respect most? Least?
3. How will these qualities in others affect your counseling?
4. Does your answer to question 2 explain each of your check marks on the list on page 50? Explain.
5. Examine the statements on page 57 made by four different clients. What is your *immediate* reaction to each? What would you say to each client? If your response is an accepting one, but your reaction to the client's statement a negative one, do you believe the client would not detect your feelings? Explain.

Bibliography

Hamrin, Shirley A., and Blanche B. Paulson, *Counseling Adolescents,* Chicago: Science Research Associates, 1950, chapter 10.

Rogers, Carl R., "The Attitude and Orientation of the Counselor in Client-Centered Therapy," *Journal of Consulting Psychology,* 13, 82-94.

Rogers, Carl R., *Client-Centered Therapy,* New York: Houghton-Mifflin Co., 1951, chapter 2.

Chapter V

THE DYNAMICS OF THE COUNSELING RELATIONSHIP

The counseling interview is a relationship between a trained specialist and a person seeking help. It is a dynamic relationship in that it precipitates change. The interaction of counselor and client in the permissive atmosphere of the interview is a moving force that produces clearer perception and more effective behavior. What does the counselor do to establish such a dynamic relationship?

The techniques in counseling are the specific skills that contribute to the process of counseling. These skills are important to counseling and the beginning counselor will want to master them. It is essential to note, however, that successful counseling is not equal to the sum of the skills the counselor can employ. Counseling is all of this—all of the skills—plus something more.

There are football players who can pass, block, kick, run, and learn signals, and yet are very mediocre players. They lack the something extra of the many good football players who with these same skills, and sometimes with fewer, can win games.

A finer analogy may be drawn between counseling and one of the arts. The portrait painter must know how to mix his oils, to apply colors to the canvas, to create the illusions of depth and perspective, and to sketch anatomical dimensions in proper proportion. Still, all of these together do not make the great artist. Rembrandt's, Van Dyke's, Monet's, and Degas' portraits possess the something-more, the essence of a personality, the feelings of the subject that the artist has captured and injected on the canvas so that the face contains the meaning of an individual.

Techniques are indispensable to the counselor, but this artist in human relations must be able to achieve the something-more. He must be able to create the climate in which the subject can "pose" naturally, and in which the counselor helps the client capture the essence of self and see it clearly. We would hazard a guess that there are few college students who could not learn the techniques of counseling. They could learn some of them as rapidly and as mechanically as one can learn to type or drive a car. The something-other is not so easily mastered. The something-other that we describe in this chapter might more accurately be called a relationship based on respect and acceptance and a sensitivity to feelings of people. Preliminary research [1,2] on the changes that occur in classes in counseling suggests that this something more can be learned in certain types of classroom experience. Further research is now under way.[3] Tentatively we may say that these learnings can be acquired but that they are so much a part of the counselor's personality, his attitudes toward people and his sensitivity to their feelings that the focus in the study of counseling must be as much on the counselor as on the client. When the counselor-trainee understands the effect of counselor on client and client on counselor (the dynamics of the counseling relationship) and can create conditions nec-

[1] Douglas O. Blocksma as reported in Carl R. Rogers' *Client-Centered Therapy,* New York: Houghton-Mifflin, 1951, p. 452-458.

[2] Walter Lifton, *A Study of the Changes in Self-Concept and Content Knowledge in Students Taking a Course in Counseling Technique,* Unpublished Ph. D. Thesis, New York University, 1950.

[3] Walter Lifton, "A Pilot Study to Investigate the Effect of Supervision on the Empathic Ability of Counseling Trainees." Now under way at the University of Illinois

essary to achieve the goals he sets for his counseling, then he has mastered the something-more. This kind of learning is not the automatic result of a program of courses or of the successful completion of a curriculum for a graduate degree. It does not occur within a prescribed period of time. For some, it comes quickly; for others, after great effort; for still others, it never comes.

Beginners in any activity reach out for specific methods the mastery of which will lead to success. "Tell me what I must do to be a good counselor," says the graduate student, "and I'll work hard at it. What are the directions? What techniques should I practice?" If this were a skill like tennis, one could suggest that he should practice keeping his eyes on the ball, gripping the racket, swinging with proper follow-through. The directions in the study of counseling require that the learner should keep his eye on himself as well as on his client, and primarily on the relationship of the two.

If there are not the tangible techniques in counseling that are directly related to success, there is at least only one goal that the counselor-trainee need set for himself. This might almost be regarded as the formula for success in counseling, a formula applicable to all types of clients, in all types of institutions, in all situations. The formula is: *The counselor-client relationship,* based on respect for the client and sensitivity to his feelings, *that makes for client self-evaluation and client growth, equals effective counseling.*

The formula is important for techniques of the counseling interview. The desirability and usefulness of a counseling tool, a counselor statement, or a counseling plan are evaluated in terms of their contribution to this relationship. All of the techniques discussed in this and the next chapter are means of implementing the counselor's purpose of creating the climate in which the client can achieve self-understanding through the efforts of both of them in a mutual undertaking.

Perhaps you wonder why all of this theorizing about a relationship. A student comes in and asks for sex information or for help in relieving a headache. Why not give it to him right off? Why fuss about his attitudes and feelings, or those of the counselor, or about a warm accepting relationship? Tell him the facts, give him a book, or have the nurse give him an aspirin.

There are students who can benefit from this kind of help. There are many others who come ostensibly for either of the purposes mentioned (sex information or an aspirin), but who will not be helped by the information or the pill, or at best will receive only temporary relief. Many adolescents and adults have inadequate or distorted knowledge of sex, but their inefficient behavior stems not from ignorance but from their attitudes toward sex. No amount of facts will by itself alter the feelings and sexual behavior of the person who has learned to associate sex with sin.

The health counselor recognizes causes of varied depth of emotional involvement in the problem of the client. At one extreme is the client who comes for information on the desirable flexibility of tooth brush bristle for her gums, and who makes it clear to the counselor that she truly desires no more than that. At the other extreme is the girl of high academic standing who is in mortal fear of a dentist and refuses to get dental treatment though her teeth are rapidly deteriorating. Fortunately for the health counselor, most of his clients are somewhere between these two. So long as attitudes and feelings are involved in the problem, and they are in this middle zone, the counselor who wishes to be effective must understand the dynamics of the counseling relationship.

On completion of the freshman physical examination in one university health center, each student is given an opportunity for a conference with the coordinator who is a physician. Almost invariably the student starts the conference with a statement, such as, "I just wanted to know about my X-ray." The physician-health counselor provides the information or interpretation implied in the question, using this initial exchange to develop a warm, permissive psychological climate. The physician encourages the student to react to the facts presented, to raise further questions or to introduce any health problems. In ninety percent of the cases the student utilizes this additional opportunity. Sometimes he says, "I'd like to know more about . . ."; or he will say, "I do wonder about something; in fact I'm a little worried. I don't seem to be able to concentrate when I sit down to study. But I guess that's not your problem."

Of course this *is* the physician-health counselor problem, even if at the end of this or a subsequent interview the counselor and client will agree on referral to another specialist. Note that this physician helps students by assuming that they may have much more of a problem than is implied in their initial question or request. This physician regards the counseling relationship as essential to his health counseling function.

We are devoting the remainder of this chapter to a detailed case history of James Doe. We can best understand the dynamics of the counseling relationship when we see them in terms of an individual. Not until we know the life history and the meanings that a client brings to the interview can we appreciate the consequences of various counselor attitudes and counseling techniques.

This study of James Doe will also indicate the process by which people learn disabling attitudes toward themselves and their environment, attitudes that make them so inefficient that they must seek help. This case will be used for illustrative purposes in Chapters VI and VII.

Portrait of the Client

Who is this person that sits facing us, this person whom we are seeking to help? What life experiences have made him what he is? What is he now, this very moment we begin to work with him?

What he is determines what we shall do in the interview.

The rationale for the counseling procedure is found in large measure in the client's attitudes toward the counselor at the moment the relationship commences.

Look at a composite picture of the client, Jim Doe. No two clients are exactly alike, but all clients will have experienced some of the pressures of development, for they are a part of the process of growing up in our culture.

John and Mary Doe told their friends and relatives that they were going to have a baby. They enjoyed the good wishes of their friends, and Mrs. Doe achieved satisfaction carrying out what she had learned as a necessary part of woman's role in life. She was not entirely happy about having the baby. She enjoyed her job at the office and was due for a long desired promotion. Furthermore, she had an occasional doubt about the wisdom of her choice of a husband, John Doe, who came from a cultural group of lower status in the community than hers. Pregnancy provided a finality to the marital compact that she did not feel before, and whenever she saw her husband as a poor choice she perceived the pregnancy as a bar to her freedom. Now she was indissolubly tied to him.

Yet, it was her own doing that she was in this situation, her own and her mother's, too. She thought at times that it was mostly her mother's fault. Her mother had inadvertently overheard an argument between her and her husband, John Doe, when Mrs. Doe had blurted out in anger that the wisest thing for her to do was to divorce John. Her mother intimated that John was not entirely at fault in the argument. She pictured for Mary the degrading publicity that would ensue. They would all be stigmatized by the scandal and Mary would be a divorcee. "Your father and I wouldn't even be spared," her mother added. The conversation ended with Mary in tears and her mother whispering to her, "Maybe having a little one will fix things for you, dear. Your father and I would be so happy."

Mary felt she would never be free from John if her child continued to live. These culturally created components of her pregnancy put an additional strain on her system, causing nausea and vomiting to a greater degree than occurs in the average pregnancy. The pregnancy continued successfully and in due time James was born, a healthy, active child.

Mr. Doe had been happier during the past nine months than ever before. He had never been fully relaxed with his wife. Without being able to understand the reason, and without even feeling sure of it, he had sensed at times that his wife was annoyed with him and resisted attentions. He would forget this during their happier moments, when her dissatisfaction would evaporate in the face of love. However, his feelings of being rejected by her would return. He would sulk and be irritable, as he had learned to behave when he was a boy, and they would argue. This served to reinforce her feelings of dissatisfaction which would only further aggravate the differences between them.

During her pregnancy, Mrs. Doe had become more dependent on her husband. He was the family's breadwinner, and he enjoyed this role. He sensed her increased desire for attention and affection and responded to it. This was married life as he had always visualized it! It satisfied his deepest needs. He felt important, wanted, attractive to his wife and adequate for marriage.

His earnings were only sufficient for them to get along with the essentials of living. In order to buy gifts for his wife, he dug into the savings that had been set aside for emergencies. He did this without his wife's knowledge.

What was the atmosphere into which Jim was born? What were the attitudes of his parents to him at the moment of birth? Mrs. Doe had mixed feelings. She knew that her husband was happy with the baby. She was pleased that she had kept pace with her friends, most of whom had a child, and she was especially proud that her child was a boy. She felt good that she had accomplished what her parents had hoped for. As she lay in her hospital bed, she visualized the smiles of her parents' approval, and the envy of the unmarried girls and childless wives at the office. But the thought of the months of hard work and long hours ahead distressed her.

When she thought of her husband's loving care, tenderness, and passion of the preceding months, her body felt warm and glowing. Then came the thought of his family, visiting now more often than before, and she was annoyed and resentful. She was part of them now for good and she did not want that. She despised them. And this child was part of them, had their blood in his veins. "I'm his servant and slave now. No more freedom to go to the office to get my own salary check and feel that I'm buying my clothes. I despise his son too. . . . No! what an awful thought! I really love him. I'll take such good care of him. He'll be healthy and strong. He must be!"

Mr. Doe was flushed with joy. His fears that the marriage would collapse were almost entirely allayed during the pregnancy. Every aspect of their social and sexual relationship had improved. In his mind the great improvement in his life was associated with one event, the conception of his child, and even before Jim's birth, his father was determined to repay him by making life as pleasant as possible for him.

Jim's early life was a thoroughly organized one. His mother raised him scientifically. He ate and slept regularly, according to the prescribed hours. Mrs. Doe was proud that her boy gained weight as scheduled and that people admired his good looks. Immersed as she was in household tasks, she felt less dependent on her husband for company and for affection. When Jim was too demanding she saw his father's features in his face and was annoyed.

Mr. Doe sensed a change in their relationship. His wife was too busy now for the moments of affection. "Your son doesn't give us time for that any more," she said. Mr. Doe perceived his son as a rival. The little boy whom he loved because he had brought more genuine sense of love into his life had robbed him of the love, and feelings of hate came threateningly close to his consciousness. Mr. Doe could not face these feelings. He could only love his child and his wife.

The strong feelings of hatred were buried in both of them, but they could not remain unexpressed. They had to be vented in some form or other. And Jim felt them as he learned in this atmosphere of love and repressed hate. The psychological climate of the home gave meaning to himself, to man and male figures, as symbolized by his father, and to woman and female figures, as symbolized by his mother. What James will become had been determined to a substantial degree by the time he entered the world. His inheritance and constitutional make-up partly determined this. More influential were the attitudes of those in his world, the people with whom he spent his life and from whom he learned his worth, his adequacy, his attractiveness. He learned very largely from them what to value in life.

For the infant, early learnings of the world occur at a warm, soft breast, or in the warmth of the mother's arms as she bottle-feeds her baby and holds him for hours during the day. Not so with Jim. His feedings were as efficiently organized as the house cleaning and dishwashing. He must eat the proper amount at the proper time. No one must be nearby for fear of disturbing him. Kissing and holding him were restricted because of the danger of infection. Mr. Doe disapproved of these restrictions, not so much because his folks were embittered by his wife's hiding the child when they came, but because he wanted to hold his son and play with him. On the two occasions that he rebelled and held the child contrary to his wife's wishes, Jim cried when he returned him to the crib. His wife's warning that he would spoil the child seemed to be materializing and her sharp rebukes and grim forebodings were sufficient to break his rebellion almost at its inception.

When Jim began to cry for long periods without apparent cause, Mrs. Doe consulted a pediatrician. The doctor advised her to mother the baby more, explaining the importance of it. Mrs. Doe decided to find a more scientific physician who would not try to cloak his ignorance of the child's illness or nutritional deficiency by such a tale. It was especially difficult to accept such a prescription because her mother-in-law had urged her to hold the baby more.

When a second pediatrician gave her the same advice, she scheduled two fifteen-minute mothering sessions during which she dutifully held the baby, wearing a mask to protect the infant from infection.

Now Jim was walking and talking. He had learned that to be a good boy, he must keep to a schedule. When he failed to be hungry at meal time he was naughty. When he did not defecate at training time he was naughty. He learned about food and sleep and health in much the same way.

The three Does were eating breakfast. Jim was now three. He saw fruit juice and hot cereal before him. He took his spoon and brought a spoonful of the cereal to his mouth.

"No, Jim, your fruit juice first," his mother said.

"First cereal!" he answered and quickly bolted the cereal into his mouth.

"On an empty stomach we drink our fruit juice first, you naughty boy!" She pulled the bowl away from him.

"I want my cereal," he cried and ran to his mother's place to reach for it. She held him off and said as she tried to control her temper, "Go back to your seat and drink your juice or you'll catch a cold. Your friend Joey down the block had to stay in bed all week because he didn't listen to his mommy and didn't eat and drink good things."

"I want my cereal," he cried and lunged for it. Mrs. Doe pushed him aside.

"You bad boy, Mommy doesn't love a bad boy."

Jim hit her with his tiny fist and she said: "You bad boy, to hit your mother! Good boys don't hit their mommys. They listen to their mommys and eat nicely and grow up big and strong."

Jim ran out of the room and cried. He was bad. His mother said so. Later his mother came to him. He was still sniffling. "Look, your nose is stuffed, you're catching cold because you don't drink your juice and listen to mommy. Listen to your mommy, honey, and you will be a good boy and you won't get sick. Mommy will love her good boy."

Jim learned that he could have his mother's love if he was a good boy, and that to be a good boy he had to eat the foods that kept him from getting sick. Bad boys did not eat right. Bad boys got sick.

Mrs. Doe sometimes had thoughts that were terrible to her. She would think how wonderful it would be if she could be working again. That would mean having no child. How awful to think of that, she felt. A good mother does not have such ideas, and she pushed them out of her mind. At times like that she would want to do something for Jim, such as building his blocks for him, or completing his jig-saw puzzle.

Some nights she would have horrible dreams about Jim. She pictured him lying in bed suffocated by his covers, or lying on the road crushed by a car. The more she had these dreams the more she wanted to do things for her son. Until he was five he often resisted bitterly, wanting to do many things himself. But as he grew older he submitted to her wishes, allowed her to make his decisions, and had no opportunity to learn to do things for himself. Soon he depended entirely on her. Mother was a person who was always there to do things for you. Mother, a woman, was the person to whom you turned to make up your mind for you. Women make up your mind for you.

Jim learned from his father, too. His father played with him, threw him in the air, carried him on his back. There were times when he did not like his father. Once when he was three, his parents argued at supper. After supper, Jim tried to get his father to play with him as he often did before bed. His father was reading the newspaper. Jim hit the newspaper and his father, in a rage, yelled, grabbed him up in his arms, and spanked him hard. This happened on several occasions.

Another evening, when Mr. Doe returned from work his wife told him that Jim, now four, was bad. He had sneaked into the pantry, taken cookies from the shelf, and eaten half the box just an hour before supper. He had left crumbs all over the floor and had upset the pantry. She was very emotional as she talked and Mr. Doe was disturbed by it.

"Punish him!" she shouted. "Punish that bad boy so that he'll learn once and for all who's boss in this house!" To her Jim had committed the double crime of eating between meals and of soiling the impeccably organized and gleaming house.

"Why don't *you* punish him?" he asked nervously, wanting to avoid a scene, yet fearing one.

"Aren't you his father? When are you going to begin to train him?" She talked loud and fast. Jim was frightened. He ran into the living room and hid behind the sofa. He could still hear the heated exchange.

"Well, are you going after him, or don't you see anything wrong in this? Do you want him to be as crude and unmannered as the Doe's?" She taunted him. He felt like striking her, but instead he ran into the living room.

Jim saw his father's big body come reaching down for him; he saw his father's bloodshot eyes and heard his breathing. Jim was frightened and he shrieked. He screamed as his father beat him and beat him until Mrs. Doe pulled the child away and took him into his room.

Jim did not trust his father. Not knowing what to expect from him, he avoided his father.

Later when Jim was in the first grade in school, the principal came into the room to observe the teaching. As he came near Jim, the boy began to cry and ran out of the room. When the teacher recounted this to Mrs. Doe, she said: "Funny, he acted the same way when we took him to the doctor, a year ago. It's just that he's afraid of strangers. He'll grow out of it."

Jim had learned to be afraid of his father, a man. He reacted with fear to those who were father-figures, to other men. In their presence he experienced anxiety; his body behaved as if it were confronted with a fearful situation, yet he could not rationally identify fear-provoking stimuli.

The years have passed and Jim is now 16 years old, a sophomore in high school. His home-room teacher notifies you, the health counselor, in an anecdotal report, that after a class discussion on the kind of help people sometimes need and the services available in the school, he asked if he could see you. The teacher reports that he daydreams a great deal and remains aloof from the other students. He recently dropped most of his extra-curricular activities.

Jim asks for an appointment and you arrange to see him during one of his free periods.

It will be profitable for you to think through the following questions before going on to the next chapter. This will give you an opportunity to compare your plan of action with that described later. Your plan will be based on the meanings which you have learned to give to "mother," "father," "son," Jim, a person with Jim's symptoms, an interview, and your role as a counselor.

Questions

1. What would you expect Jim's reactions to be to a female counselor? To a male counselor?
2. Why would you expect such reactions?
3. What effects would these reactions have on the interview?
4. How would you deal with these reactions?
5. What preparation, if any, would you make prior to the interview? Why?
6. What would you hope to accomplish in the first interview?
7. Ordinarily would you, the counselor, be familiar with these attitudes of Jim? Would they be available, for example, in the cumulative record?
8. What are the implications of your answers to question 7 for methods of counseling?
9. As health counselor what would you have done if, after learning of Jim's withdrawing behavior, he had not come voluntarily for counseling?

Bibliography

Cameron, Norman, *The Psychology of Behavior Disorders, A Biosocial Interpretation,* New York: Houghton-Mifflin Co., 1947. See chapter 2 for clear statement on the development of personality; also chapters 3 to 6.

Hamrin, Shirley A., and Blanche B. Paulson, *Counseling Adolescents,* Chicago: Science Research Associates, 1950, chapters 1 and 2.

Snygg, Donald, and Arthur W. Combs, *Individual Behavior, A New Frame of Reference for Psychology,* New York: Harper and Bros., 1949, chapters 2 to 8.

CHAPTER VI

TECHNIQUES OF PROMOTING THE DYNAMIC COUNSELING RELATIONSHIP

Jim comes to your office. He is unhappy and insecure. He is defensive, worried, and suspicious of you. Not only is there something bothering him, which has led him to seek help, but now something more has been added: YOU. He is going to you because he wants help. But you are still a stranger and a school official. There is something new, strange, and threatening in this.

We turn now to a discussion of techniques that can be employed to change these attitudes toward you, the counselor, and to promote the kind of relationship that will enable Jim to come to grips with his problem. These are the primary techniques in health counseling. They are techniques only in the sense that analysis[1] of the dynamic counseling relationship reveals them to be characteristics of counselor behavior. Actually they are methods used by counselors to implement their belief in the client's capacity to develop new meanings more in accord with reality; and their desire for the client to come to grips with his problem as he sees it in a permissive atmosphere. We repeat again that the techniques are mean-

[1] Julius Seeman, "A Study of the Process of Nondirective Therapy," *Journal of Counseling Psychology,* 13, 157-168 (1949).

ingless except within the context of the attitudes which they are intended to implement.

Rapport

So long as Jim continues to feel as he does at the very moment he comes to your office or an empty classroom, you will make no progress in counseling. You, therefore, establish as your first goal a change in his attitudes toward you. This is the groundwork for any further steps in counseling. Without this firm foundation, anything that transpires between counselor and client is not realistic. The client will say only what he feels free to say in a threatening situation. He will not talk of the things that worry him, especially if these usually bring forth a response of disapproval. He will react to you as he does to other strange adults. If you are a man, Jim will be even more fearful, and if a woman, his fear will be combined with an expectancy of help.

The first goal is essential in the good counseling interviews in every institution, under all circumstances, with every problem, whether the client is an alcoholic, a sexual deviant, a patient with psychosomatic symptoms, an amputee, or a school girl or boy disturbed by the first evidences of adolescence. This first step is frequently called establishing rapport.

Rapport, a word taken from the French, is one of the most widely used and misused terms in discussions on counseling. Webster defines it as follows: "1. Relation; especially, relation characterized by harmony, conformity, accord, or affinity; used especially in the phrase *in rapport* or *en rapport* . . . in an intimate or harmonious relation; as applied to people, having a close understanding or working in mutual dependence."

A sympathetic, harmonious relationship is built on trust. Jim must feel from the words of the counselor and especially from his behavior that he is not going to be judged, criticized, condemned, or falsely praised; that he is going to receive help only if he wants it.

The counselor must create the psychological climate in

which Jim can feel this way. Such a counselor must be, as one writer[2] put it, "warmly feeling and coldly reasoning." He must be able to "feel with" Jim so that he can share his feelings and understand them, yet he must be able to remain sufficiently aloof to recognize from verbalizations and bodily reactions the nature of Jim's feelings.

Rapport is a primary goal and the first consideration in counseling, yet it is not completed by a single act, nor within any time limit. It must persist throughout the counseling relationship, and the wisdom of the counselor's behavior may be evaluated in terms of its effect on rapport. Should I listen or should I speak? Should I respond to a feeling or should I question him? Should I ask about his parents, or about his attitudes toward girls? Should I call on his parents and speak with his teachers? These and other questions may be answered in terms of the effect of each of the alternatives on Jim's feelings toward the counseling and the counselor.

Rapport is sometimes established by finding and talking about some subject congenial to the client, such as a membership in the Scouts, interest in basketball or art. Surely, this may contribute to thawing out Jim and making him feel at ease. But this is just the start; the counselor has hardly begun. How he reacts toward the client when the client talks about his problem, himself and others, when he shows that his values are different from those of the counselor and of others, is the crucial point in the development of rapport. To imply in an initial exchange about a hobby that Jim can have some trust and then to criticize Jim when he begins to talk about his attitudes toward his father is to make him even more threatened, more defensive, and to impair the relationship seriously. Such a procedure might be compared with that of the teacher who tells students that they may talk freely, but then criticizes them for disagreeing with his point of view.

In some of the following paragraphs, we shall examine the

[2] Franklin Keller, in Foreword to Robert Hoppock's *Job Satisfaction,* New York: Harper and Bros., 1935.

concept of rapport, with its various facets, to recognize the components of the relationship. These components are so interrelated that the distinctions implied in their separate labels are purely academic.

Warmth

The warmly feeling counselor is the kind of person who makes the client feel welcome and comfortable. Many women working as receptionists have that quality; some of them, however, create by their brusqueness or indifference a frigid atmosphere in which one feels unwelcome and uncomfortable. Differences of this kind are evident among bus drivers, postal clerks, unemployment insurance interviewers, teachers, students, physicians, nurses, psychologists, health specialists, counselors, and others.

QUESTIONS

1. Recall an experience you have had with the "cold" kind of person. What were your feelings toward this person? What other feelings did you have?
2. Recall an experience with a "warm" person and make the same analysis of your feelings.
3. In what category would you place yourself?
4. What characteristics do you have of warmth to people? of coldness to people?
5. Are there certain categories of people toward whom you are consistently warm or cold?

Permissiveness

The counselor allows the client to say anything he wants to say. Jim would be free to express the deepest hatred for his father, resentment toward his mother, suspicion and fear of the counselor. He would be free to talk uninhibitedly of religion, education, sex, himself, the counselor, good or poor health habits, the effectiveness of the counseling. If a permissive atmosphere did not prevail, Jim could not begin to express, perhaps for the first time in his life, the deeply buried feelings that rankled in him and shaped his attitudes toward other people and are the source of his present problem. When the counselor creates this atmosphere he provides the client with emotional release. This catharsis, as it is called, is a positive step toward facing realities more objectively. Its value lies not only in the release of strongly colored feelings, but also in the fact that the counselor's acceptance of the feelings puts a new cast on them for the client.

In this atmosphere, the client would also be free to decide what is important for him to discuss with the counselor and what to avoid. He would feel that he has the right to regard the counseling as worthless and to terminate it when he desires. He would feel free to choose for himself the course that his life is to take.[3,4]

How does the counselor succeed in creating this permissiveness? (1) He must like people and gain satisfaction from counseling with them. (2) He must be unthreatened and unshaken by the client's doubts of his ability to help. (3) He must be able to accept without personal disturbance and dis-

[3] "It has seemed clear, from our clinical experience as well as our research, that when the counselor perceives and accepts the client as he is, when he lays aside all evaluation and enters into the perceptual frame of reference of the client, he frees the client to explore his life and experience anew, frees him to perceive in that experience new meanings and new goals. But is the therapist willing to give the client full freedom as to outcomes? Is he genuinely willing for the client to organize and direct his life? Is he willing for him to choose goals that are social or antisocial, moral or immoral? Even more difficult, is he willing for the client to choose regression rather than growth or maturity? to choose neuroticism rather than mental health? to choose to reject help rather than accept it? to choose death rather than life? To me it appears that only as the therapist is completely willing that *any* outcome, any direction, may be chosen—only then does he realize the vital strength of the capacity and potentiality of the individual for constructive action. It is as he is willing for death to be the choice, that life is chosen, for neuroticism to be the choice that a healthy normality is chosen. The more completely he acts upon his central hypothesis the more convincing is the evidence that the hypothesis is correct." Rogers, Carl R. "The Attitude and Orientation of the Counselor in Client-Centered Therapy." *Journal of Consulting Psychology*, p. 94, 13 (April, 1949).

[4] For a vivid example of the impact of permissiveness and freedom of choice see Act V of Henrik Ibsen's *The Lady From the Sea*.

play of shock the client's descriptions of behavior and expressions of feeling, no matter how sordid, perverted, or sacrilegious.

Acceptance

Jim would feel comfortable not only because he found the counselor warm and the atmosphere permissive, but also because the counselor accepted all his feelings. He did not have to guard against saying the wrong thing. This person listening to him so intently was no censor. He was not disapproving nor approving his words. Whatever idea he thought, whatever feeling he felt, Jim could express them to this person when he felt ready to do so.

Client-directed

Despite his experience, training, and understanding of human behavior, the counselor does not lecture, persuade, or prescribe. It would be more accurate to say that he avoids these approaches *because* of his understanding of human behavior.

Jim's attitudes toward people and health stem from his experiences which have given distorted meanings to them. Woman is a person who handles all problems for a fellow. This meaning of Jim's cannot be changed by any of the methods just mentioned. Nobody can be forced to stop having certain thoughts. Perhaps he can be made to feel guilty or stupid for having them, but this will only make him unhappier without altering the meanings.

The counselor is aware that he himself does not know the cause of Jim's trouble and should not act as if he did. He knows that his client has learned certain attitudes toward himself and his parents, friends, teachers, and school that are disabling. His primary task is not in finding the causes, but in enabling Jim to learn new attitudes. Sometimes the counselor regards himself unqualified or otherwise unprepared to accomplish this. In this case, the goal for Jim remains unchanged. The counselor adds an intermediary one: to create the rapport that will lead Jim to say, "Yes I do want help. Since you say you are not qualified, then I would like someone who is as nice as you are, but who is qualified."

Structuring

This is still another aspect of the relationship. We feel comfortable in a situation when we know the purpose of our being there and the role we are to play. The client who goes to the counselor of his own volition knows the purposes but not his role. The unmotivated client, who has been asked to come, knows neither.

When Jim comes to the office, he wonders what will happen. What will this stranger they call "counselor" do and say? What will he expect of me? What will he do if I say the wrong thing?

The threat and uncertainty of the counseling situation are partly allayed when the client becomes familiar with his role and the counselor's in this new relationship. Note how the counselor starts the interview, as Jim appears in the office doorway:

> *Counselor* (a smile on his face): Hello, Jim, please come in.
>
> *Jim:* Hello (walks timidly toward the counselor's desk).
>
> *Counselor:* Won't you sit down? This isn't the softest of chairs, but it's comfortable. (Places the chair facing his, both on the same side of the desk.)
>
> *Jim:* Thanks.
>
> *Counselor:* Would you like to tell me what it is that brought you here?

What is the meaning of this question to Jim?

The counselor is telling him to start wherever he wishes. He is not asking specific questions. It is for Jim to take the responsibility for the direction of the interview. As the interview proceeds Jim recognizes the nature of this relationship

If he had difficulty in accepting it and were to ask the counselor to question him, he would receive the following kind of response:

> *Counselor*: Suppose you talk about what you want to. My job is to understand whatever problems you raise. Then maybe the two of us together will see things work out. If you can't think of anything to say, or prefer not to talk for a while, that's perfectly all right.

Whether or not the structure of the interview is verbally described to the client, what is more important is the structuring that stems from the behavior of the counselor and his attitudes toward the client. Without uttering a word about it, a counselor can let it be known that he is going to dominate the interview, that he is going to point out the direction; likewise, he can indicate by his behavior that he expects the client to assume the initiative in raising problems and pointing the direction. The client learns very soon that in counseling, he responds as the counselor does. The client recognizes the cues from the counselor that he should lead the way or that he should follow, that he should talk freely about any subject, any feelings, or that he should be on guard against criticism.

The problems of counseling are doubly compounded when working with an unmotivated person. The counselor can inform him of the services available and inform him by his attitudes and manner that it is for the client to decide whether or not to use these services. The counselor assumes that if the unmotivated client feels the interest and the respect of the counselor, he may want help, now or in the future. He also assumes that while he can bring the client to his office, he cannot forcibly make him change the distorted meanings that constitute his outlook on life. He knows he cannot force the highly self-conscious amputee to eliminate these feelings. If and when the unmotivated client chooses to come for counseling, the counselor must inform him, by his behavior much more than by his words, that the issues they will deal with in the interviews will be those which the client wishes to raise.

The counseling relationship based on warmth, permissiveness, acceptance, and understanding of the client-directed role can be a fruitful one. These characteristics must be present throughout the counseling, not just in the first ten minutes or in the first interview. If these characteristics of rapport are compatible with the counselor's personality, his outlook on life, his attitudes toward people, they will inevitably be present in all of his professional activities.

Dealing with the Problem

This heading is misleading for it implies that we have not yet discussed the means of dealing with problems. Actually, when the counselor creates rapport, he is enabling the two of them, client and counselor, to deal with the problem.

Accepting the Client's Feelings of Self and the Problem

Our client, Jim, has come into our office. He is now somewhat at ease, and is talking. His speech is halting and slightly confused, as he is torn with ambivalent feelings about expressing his intimate thoughts, and as he struggles to verbalize feelings that have never been expressed. After about five minutes, he says:

> *Jim:* I wonder if you can help me. I've got a problem. It's my face. All the acne. I hate it.

How will you, the counselor, respond? Let us examine the various possible responses.

> *Counselor 1:* Sure I can help you. The first thing to do is to stop worrying about it. It's not nearly as bad as you think it is. I hardly noticed it until you mentioned it.

Would you give this kind of response? Why?

We have noticed that Jim, like all of us, has developed from his experience personal meanings about himself, his parents, people, health. Through our priviliged genetic study, we have information about Jim that counselors do not have prior to counseling. We know that acne must have some special meaning for him that it may not have for other people. The response of counselor 1 as much as says to Jim: "Turn off your feelings; they are wrong. Although your whole life has made you feel this way, your feelings are wrong and I advise you to change them. If you had not pointed it out I would hardly have taken notice."

Perhaps you can evaluate the wisdom of this response by recalling a comparable experience of your own when someone told you there was no cause for worry. Did it end your worries?

Physicians are familiar with the patient who is ridden with fears of some disease. No matter how often a thorough examination gives negative results, his anxieties persist, and he goes from physician to physician for confirmation of something that his experiences convince him must be true. Sometimes denial of one disease will only lead him to fix on another. Neither ignorance, nor perversity, nor dishonesty is responsible for this irrational behavior. It is a product of the patient's life experiences and is entirely consistent with the lessons he has learned about himself. Only when the *meanings* he has acquired have been changed and made more in accord with objective reality will his *behavior* be altered. These meanings can be changed by manipulating an individual's environment, as, for example, by providing a child with the experience of success. This will be discussed in the next chapter. We are considering in this chapter changes in meanings brought about by counseling with the motivated client.

Some of Jim's most emotional experiences have been related to health and the evil of ill health. The words of a counselor will not erase these life experiences. On the contrary, they will lead Jim to decide that this counselor does not understand and will lead to loss of confidence in him. At best, the counselor's reassurance may give Jim a temporary lift that will evaporate within a few hours or days, when *his* understandings—not the counselor's—will interpret the experiences he has, the evidences he sees in the behavior of others that his acne is hateful and that it is a problem.

Counselor 1's response is a poor one: It tells Jim that his feelings are wrong, but makes no attempt to help Jim change the meanings that create the feelings. It raises doubt in the client concerning the counselor's judgment; it undermines rapport because the client's own feelings are challenged at the outset; it informs the client that the counselor believes himself to be an oracle with the answers to all of life's problems.

> *Counselor 2:* Sure I can help you, Jim. Why that's not such a terrible problem. Look, here's what we can do. I'll arrange for you to see the school doctor. He will give you treatments that will probably clear up the acne.

Would you give this kind of response? Why?

This counselor has decided in a flash that acne is the only problem and that dealing with the acne is equivalent to dealing with Jim's problem. We who know Jim's personal history, as no counselor can know it prior to counseling, are aware that his strong reactions to the acne are bound up with the attitudes he learned from his mother about the evils of ill health. A discerning counselor, even if he is not familiar with Jim's background, would recognize in the client's behavior, in the interview, something more serious than just the acne. He would not know the importance of the acne in reinforcing Jim's shyness and fear, but he would recognize the significance of Jim's feelings to his present adjustment. He would, therefore, place the focus on these feelings.

Counselor 2 does at least accept Jim's feelings and wants to be helpful. His error is in assuming that Jim knows precisely what is troubling him when he enters and, if he does know, that he is prepared to talk about it to him, a stranger. Counselor 2 has decided at once that he knows the problem and its solution. This is not to imply that medical treatment for Jim is undesirable; it implies only that it may not be, and we know it is not the entire answer to Jim's problems; that it is premature for the counselor to introduce it for he cuts off the client's opportunity to go on to examine himself, to free himself of some of his feelings; and it informs Jim that the counselor knows the problem and will cure it for Jim. Thus, this boy, trained to be highly dependent on his mother, has now found another person who takes over responsibility for him.

> *Counselor 3:* You'll have to tell me more about it, Jim. How much candy do you eat? (This is followed by questions on sleep, exercise, relaxation, social life, and other factors.)

Would you give this kind of response? Why?

Counselor 3 has also assumed that Jim's problem is acne. Then, by the manner in which he conducts the interview, he informs his client that from now on he can sit back and relax and allow the counselor to discover the cause of his difficulties and to cure them.

We know that this approach will not be effective. The battery of questions about his health will probably reveal good health practices. Even if it should disclose that Jim is not getting enough sleep, the counselor's admonition to get more sleep would not change the meanings Jim has acquired that have made acne something much more than just a blemished complexion.

> *Counselor 4:* You're very much upset by the looks of your face.

Would you give this kind of response? Why?

This response of Counselor 4 says to Jim: this is your feeling, is it not? I accept it. Feel free to go on talking some more, in the direction you want to go, for it is you—not I—who can know what is important. At the moment acne and your face are important to you. I may wonder whether this is your real problem. I may know some ways of dealing with the acne. I may be curious about your physical and mental hygiene, but I believe that the shortest route to overcoming your difficulties is the route that you choose to travel. I want you, Jim, to know that this counseling is a shared responsibility. I respect your integrity as an individual and restore to you the opportunity to gain the self-respect that comes from the ability to assume responsibility for one's life, to direct the course of one's life and to make decisions. Whatever it has been that has led you to develop meanings about yourself and your health that set you apart from others (the counselor does not have the benefit of Jim's personal life that we have), I give you now—either through me or through another professional worker—the opportunity to develop meanings about yourself and your world that are more in accord with the realities of your life. I cannot do this for you. I cannot convert new meanings from old. If I make such a claim, I am either a charlatan or a fool. Only you can change them. I can only provide the warm human relationship and the counseling skills that will help you achieve it.

Yes, this is a great deal to deduce from a single counselor response. But even single responses reveal much about the counselor's attitudes and his philosophy of counseling. Counselors are like clients in at least one respect: They also act in terms of the meanings they have attached to themselves and their world. Counselor 1 perceives his role as one of showing the bright side of things. The meaning of counseling for him is to make light of anything that concerns the client, at least if it does not appear to be significant in his, the counselor's eyes. Perhaps this counselor has learned that when something makes you unhappy, deny its existence, and you will be happy again. He carries this attitude into counseling.

To Counselor 2, counseling means doing something to the client. It means accepting physical symptoms as indicators of the problem and disregarding the strong feelings expressed. Counseling means hearing the complaint and directing the client to the solution.

To Counselor 3, counseling is the process of uncovering, by probing questions and sometimes by various sleuthlike methods, the cause of the symptoms. His is the process of diagnosing and then of prescribing, as for example, "you should get more sleep," or "you should go out with girls." The meaning of the counselor's role for him is that of an expert who can find the maladjustment, as a physician finds an infection, and then prescribe the measures that will eliminate it. But will prescriptions change meanings? Will Jim learn to see himself differently, to regard himself with greater esteem, to feel more liked and loved if he joins various school activities? Or is it likely that with his present outlook on himself unchanged, he may well meet with further evidence, for him, of his unattractiveness to others, of being unloved, and of being inept in social situations? Will Jim be motivated to become more of a social being when the counselor points out that what he needs to relieve him of his feelings of being unliked and unattractive is more participation in extracurricular activities?

Counselor 4 regards clients as people who have acquired meanings that make living inefficient because they are distortions of the realities of their lives. Behavior to him is a function of these personal meanings, and can be changed only by a reorganization of these meanings. A counselor, to him, is a person who can only provide the permissive, accepting atmosphere in which Jim can learn to explore the values he has attached to himself, to others, to his activities, and to change them so that they are more in accord with reality.

CLARIFYING THE CLIENT'S FEELINGS

What good does counselor 4's response do? Is it not the counselor's responsibility to help the client? And how can such a response be helpful? Would it not really leave the client confused, not knowing what to do next?

In making his response, the counselor is attempting to reflect Jim's feelings. "This is your feeling, as I get it," he says. "You have the right to this feeling." Jim soon comes to see that he has the right to release his feelings and to examine them without shame. This release, this emotional catharsis, is in itself beneficial. The reader may recall the satisfying experience of releasing highly pent-up feelings by telling a personal friend of socially disapproved behavior. The mere act of sharing unacceptable thoughts and feelings with another human and especially of experiencing their acceptance by the counselor makes them less offensive, and makes the individual more objective in evaluating them.

Thus, Jim has a chance to examine his attitudes and meanings toward his parents, his self, health, and any other phenomena of his experience, and then to change them as he comes to see that other meanings are more appropriate. For example, as his attitudes toward health become clearer to him, he recognizes that health and morals have somehow become confused. He sees that acne has become confused with the feeling of being bad. Now he changes the meaning of acne. It is a skin blemish. He wants to eliminate it if he can, and he is prepared for medical treatment.

Whether cleared up or not, acne will no longer interfere, to the same intense degree, with his social relations and with his general living efficiency. Now that it has a different meaning, a meaning with lesser weight or value, its effect on his behavior is proportionately diminished.

In the presence of his classmates, he does not feel now that he shows evidence of evil on his face; he no longer feels evil because other meanings, not discussed here, have also been revised and, as a result, he can truly feel he belongs to his group.

A client may not like the counselor to remain noncommittal about his feelings. The client may prefer to have the counselor tell him what to do, for he is probably accustomed to dependent relationships which are fostered in our homes and schools. A new kind of relationship is threatening. But he also senses the counselor's genuine interest and warmth and finds support in this. As he gains success in taking responsibilities, he discovers what all children and adolescents do: that the threats of assuming responsibility and gaining independence, such as spending the first night away from home, are coupled with the joys of growing up and doing things for oneself. This success gives him more courage.

We have noted that people learn in a short time the role that is expected of them. When the counselor lets it be known by his behavior that he is going to ask questions and direct the course of the interview, the client will wait for questions and follow the counselor's leadership. When the counselor lets it be known that he is interested in whatever the client says, and that his expressions will constitute the content and determine the course of the interview, the client will take the initiative. Perhaps he will do it haltingly at first and with some discomfort, but he will do it.

Client Responsibility

As Jim begins to perceive himself differently, as his parents, his classmates, his eating habits, and other experiences take on new meanings for him, he changes his behavior. He changes it because he wants to change it, because it makes sense to him now to change it, not because he is ordered, urged, or begged to change it. Now Jim wants to join with others in play and work, because he perceives himself as acceptable to others. He wants medical treatment. He wants to break loose from the stifling love of his mother and to react with less fear and more friendliness to his father.

Are all of Jim's problems solved? Are his difficulties ended? By no means! He has many battles ahead. Learning new roles in life is not easy, whether it is a new role as son or a new role as member of a peer group. The new Jim knows now what he wants and how he wants to live. He has that most dynamic human quality to achieve these goals—motivation. He is now a better integrated, a much more unified person. He has learned in counseling that he is worthy of respect, that he can deal with his problems, and he has learned mature ways of thinking about himself and his problems.

Jim has learned this new outlook because he has participated in a mature relationship in which he has replaced dependency by self-responsibility. With the drive for growth, health, and maturity no longer blocked, he can act efficiently in such a way as to satisfy his need for maintenance and enhancement of self, for the feeling of self-respect, of being liked and wanted by his peers.

What are the characteristics of the interview that promote client maturity?

(1) The client chooses the topics for discussion and determines the direction of the interview.

(2) The client makes his own decisions and charts his own plans.

(3) The client's hours and time allotment are predetermined, and are adhered to. Client tardiness and client desire to hang on to the counselor at the end of the hour are not permitted to alter these. The client learns to face himself freely (in this permissive atmosphere), but within the limitations that one finds in a social world.

(4) The counselor promotes (1) and (2), largely by being a warm, permissive, accepting person, by reflecting and clarifying the client's feelings, and fundamentally by believing that *the client,* and every individual, *has the capacity* to clear

away the blinding veils of distorted self-perception and to realign these perceptions with the realities of his life.

Some questions come to mind at this time. You may want to answer them yourself, before they are discussed in the text.

Questions

1. Is this counseling approach practical or just the pipe dream of college professors?
2. When should the counselor provide the client with information?
3. How can other members of the professional staff (in school, agency, or hospital) be utilized in counseling?
4. Can group techniques be used in working with clients like Jim?
5. In what ways is counseling unmotivated clients different from counseling motivated clients?

Exercises

I

After each client statement in the following exercise are five or six counselor responses. Explain the meaning to the client of each response, and the probable effect on him or her. Which response would you make? Why?

A disabled veteran, arm amputated three inches below the elbow, now in his first year in college comes to you, one of his instructors. After an exchange of pleasantries he says:

(1) I'm having a tough time with my work. I just can't get it done. I know I can do it, but I don't.

- (a) You feel you can and yet you don't. That's sort of inconsistent, eh? (said with a smile).
- (b) Perhaps you haven't developed good study habits. Let's talk about that.
- (c) I understand; a lot of fellows in your boat have that trouble. You're still so upset by your handicap that it's hard for you to concentrate.

(d) You're sure you can do it, but something stops you from it.
(e) It seems to me that maybe you're not motivated—maybe you're taking the wrong course.

(2) (later in interview) Do you know what it's like to choose between this (points to the half-empty sleeve) and a hook? Do you know what it's like to be stared at like a freak?
(a) I know it must be tough, but you're no freak (said very kindly).
(b) I know it's no fun, but it doesn't end life, you know.
(c) Why not look at the bright side of things? You're a good looking fellow.
(d) It's a blow to your status; you feel different.
(e) You're pretty mad about it.

A student nurse comes to you, her superior, and asks if she may talk with you. You offer her a seat. The student says, as tears well to her eyes:

(3) Miss Smith is picking on me all the time. I can't stand it any more.
(a) You're all upset by it. Please go on.
(b) I'm surprised. Miss Smith has always been fair to students.
(c) A nurse has got to learn to take orders.
(d) Is it possible that you're imagining this?
(e) Don't cry (sweetly said). Let me call Miss Smith so we can talk about it together.

(4) (later in interview) Maybe I don't belong in nursing.
(a) (kindly) Why don't you let us decide. After all, we are experienced.
(b) You're not very sure of yourself now.
(c) You wouldn't be here if you didn't.
(d) You thought Miss Smith didn't like you and it's destroyed your confidence.
(e) What do your parents think?

Male, veteran student, age 25 (1947), college sophomore:

(5) She was sick when we started to go together. Bad heart and I knew she'd never be normal. . . . (pause; speaks as if off in distance). I used to carry her upstairs when I took her to my house. But I thought she'd get stronger. God, but I loved her. What's the use of going on now?

- (a) You feel she was more important to you than anything else.
- (b) You feel it important for *me* to answer your question?
- (c) There's just nothing left to make you want to go on. Is that it?
- (d) Life must go on. Time heals the sores and we find purposes in life.
- (e) There is much use. You can dedicate your life to her, so that her life will not have been in vain.
- (f) You feel that she would have liked you to feel that way?

II

Below are thumb-nail sketches of four health-counseling cases. Play the role of the counselor, writing your response to each statement. Justify your response in terms of the effect each would be likely to have on the client. Try out your responses on a roommate or friend or classmate. Have that person read the client statements and you give your response. Later, ask the role-playing client for his reactions to you as a counselor.

John

John is a high-school junior. He is average in height and weight for his age and slender in build. His complexion is noticeably marred by acne eruptions. You know him as a bright student who excels in written work but who never talks in your class except when questioned. You have noticed that he does not get involved in the active conversations that go on before the bell. If you had been asked whether he was a happy boy, you would have said *no* unhesitantly.

Today, John lingers after class. He fumbles with his books, glances in your direction as you are working at your desk, and finally, with great effort, comes to your desk.

Counselor:
(1) *John:* I'd like to ask you something.
Counselor:
(2) *John:* I don't know if I should. It's not really about class.
Counselor:
(3) *John:* My face is a mess.
Counselor:
(4) *John:* What can I do about it?
Counselor:
(5) *John:* Girls don't want to go with a "pimple-face." I heard one of them call me that.
Counselor:
(6) *John:* I feel that . . . that nobody likes me.
Counselor:
(7) *John:* My mother knows what's best.
Counselor:
(8) *John:* Maybe I shouldn't listen to her so much.
Counselor:
(9) *John:* What can I do? Can you help me?
Counselor:

Elizabeth

Elizabeth, 14½ years old, is a 9th grade student. She is taller and physically more matured than her classmates, and is sometimes mistaken for a 17 or 18 year old. She has been a disturbing influence in your class, frequently tardy and deliberately noisy in her entrance into the classroom. She has made disparaging remarks aimed at you and at the good students in the class, and has exploited every opportunity for a "wisecrack." Other teachers have remarked that she is "a bad girl" and that she would find herself in a reform school.

You have told her privately several times during the past two months that you would be glad to talk with her. You have checked her medical record with the school nurse (no defects or history of serious illness); her academic record (average performance in elementary school, steady decline in junior high school); her psychological test record (four I.Q.'s over the past 8 years, with range of 104-108); and family information (mother at home, father owns service station, younger brother in 6th grade).

Elizabeth comes into your empty classroom at the end of the day. She stands before you now, proud and stubbornly silent. Indicate the remarks you would make in counseling this student, and the response you would expect Elizabeth to make to your first statement.

(1) *Counselor:*
Elizabeth:
Counselor:

(2) *Elizabeth:* I don't need anybody's help. I'm no mommy's boy!
Counselor:

(3) *Elizabeth:* Do you think I'm afraid of the teachers in this school? Not me!
Counselor:

(4) *Elizabeth:* You're all the same, all you teachers. (excitedly) And you're no different. You want to step on me, too. I'll bet that's why you wanted me to come here.
Counselor:

(5) *Elizabeth:* Some kids like to come to school. They say it's fun. I hate it. Why should I have to come?
Counselor:

(6) *Elizabeth:* I wish I weren't so big.
Counselor:

(7) *Elizabeth:* Friends? No, I don't have real friends. But the girls wish they were like me, especially (smiles and stares at the floor) when I wear a sweater.
Counselor:

* * *

(8) *Elizabeth:* Can you tell me . . . about what happens every month?
Counselor:

William

It is the policy in your high school that all students who either refuse to take gym or who are frequently absent from the gym class are sent to *you* (whether you are nurse, health educator, counselor, head of the physical education department, or classroom teacher).

William, a generally well-behaved tenth-grade student, has been referred to you by the gym teacher. The gym teacher explained, in a note you received a day before the boy's appointment with you, that William has been absent occasionally, tardy frequently, and that at all times when he does come, he tends to stay in the background, avoid competition and exertion. He has spoken with William, but "I have gotten nowhere. He's stubborn."

You check the records and find it unblemished except for gym. He is a "B" student, in the commercial field, rarely absent, never tardy, except in physical education. He has no record of serious illness or defect.

Now as he walks into your office (or classroom) after school, you see a fairly attractive boy, average height and weight, dressed neatly in a well-pressed suit, shirt, tie, and polished shoes. You speak first as he approaches. When he first starts to talk he is polite but unsmiling and "holding back."

(1) *Counselor:*
William: Hello, sir (or ma'm). Mr. Smith, the gym teacher, asked me to come to see you.
Counselor:

(2) *William:* I'm sort of forgetful at times. That's why I'm late for gym.
Counselor:

(3) *William:* I don't like to break rules. Honest I don't. And I don't like Mr. Smith to think I don't like him.
Counselor:

(4) *William:* How do I feel about taking gym? Well, I like all my other subjects. Don't you think a pupil's got a right to dislike one of them?
Counselor:

(5) *William:* I'm no sissy. Some of the boys think so. Just because a boy is clean doesn't make him a sissy, does it?
Counselor:

(6) *William:* Sure I like sports. I love to swim especially. That's wonderful fun.
Counselor:

(7) *William:* And I like to play ball, too. In the Spring we play softball in my neighborhood. Now sometimes we play touch football. Then I go in and bathe and we have dinner. (With a smile) Boy, you sure feel good then.
Counselor:

(8) *William:* I don't like to go to my next class sweaty and smelly.
Counselor:

Howard

The high school coach phones you, the health counselor. "We've got a ticklish problem here and thought you could help," he says. "You know Howard D——, the boy who was a star on our football team last year when he was only a sophomore. You know he's got a rheumatic heart and can't play the game again. The kid won't listen to reason, says he's got to play. Will you see him and try to knock some sense into his head?" You suggest an hour the following day.

You talk with the school nurse who confirms the diagnosis and the restriction placed on his activity by his physician. You check the nonmedical records. The boy is a slightly better than average student in the college preparatory curriculum. His best grades are in math and science. He has no extracurricular activities, no hobbies other than sports.

He comes to your office at the appointed hour. He is tense, but not shy.

(1) *Howard:* The coach told me to see you. He said you could help me.
Counselor:

(2) *Howard:* The coach said you were a good guy and that you'd help me. I want to play football and they won't let me.
Counselor:

(3) *Howard*: They say my heart's bad. They're crazy! I feel fine. I'm strong. I was sick, but I'm all better. I can run just as fast as before, and I can lift as much. Tell them to let me play.
Counselor:

(4) Howard: You're in charge of health here, aren't you? Why don't you try me out? Go ahead and test my heart.
Counselor:

(5) *Howard*: I've *got* to play. I tell you I've just got to play.
Counselor:

(6) *Howard*: What's there in life for a fella if he can't play ball?
Counselor:

(7) *Howard:* If I don't play it will be like being an invalid all my life.
Counselor:

(8) *Howard:* Maybe I'm like some of the disabled vets. My friend's brother is one. I guess he wants to live and have fun.
Counselor:

(9) *Howard:* What's there for me if I can't play?
Counselor:

Bibliography

Axline, Virginia M., *Play Therapy,* New York: Houghton Mifflin Co., 1947. The use of client-centered counseling with children, in which much of the feeling of the children is expressed in play rather than in words.

Bingham, Walter V. D., and Bruce V. Moore, *How to Interview,* New York: Harper and Bros., 1941, chapters 2, 3, and 8.

Brayfield, Arthur H., *Readings in Modern Methods of Counseling,* New York: Appleton-Century-Crofts, 1950, chapter 31, "Structuring the Counseling Relationship: A Case Report," by

Charles A. Curran; chapter 11, "The Development of Insight in a Counseling Relationship," by Carl R. Rogers; chapter 35, "An Investigation of the Nature of Nondirective Psychotherapy," by William U. Snyder; chapter 36, Self-Reference in Counseling Interviews," by Victor C. Raimy; chapter 37, "The Role of Client Talk in the Counseling Interview," by Earl F. Carnes and Francis P. Robinson.

Garrett, Annette, *Interviewing, Its Principles and Methods,* New York: Family Welfare Association of America, 1942.

Porter, E. H., Jr., *An Introduction to Therapeutic Counseling,* New York: Houghton Mifflin Co., 1950. A valuable book in the training of the counselor, including discussion of the various types of problems that confront the counselor, and many exercises.

Rogers, Carl R., *Counseling and Psychotherapy,* New York: Houghton Mifflin Co., 1942, chapter 4 and part III.

Rogers, Carl R., *Client-Centered Therapy,* New York: Houghton Mifflin Co., 1951, chapters 3 and 4; chapter 6, "Play Therapy," by Elaine Dorfman.

Snyder, W. U., *Casebook of Nondirective Counseling,* New York: Houghton Mifflin Co., 1947.

Snygg, Donald, and Arthur W. Combs, *Individual Behavior, A New Frame of Reference for Psychology,* New York: Harper and Bros., 1949, chapter 14.

Chapter VII

THE CASE WORK APPROACH

In this chapter, we discuss the methods used by counselors in helping the unmotivated client. By case work, we mean the process of studying the maladjusted individual to determine the changes necessary in the individual's status or environment to produce changes in his meanings and his behavior. We call it the case-work approach to differentiate these functions of the counselor from those that rely largely on the counseling interview. The counselor's destination remains the same; only his route is different.

We will also discuss the use of various group procedures. These are valuable in working with individuals unmotivated for counseling. Since they are also effective preventive measures for all students who are daily experiencing constitutional and social changes, their varied uses will be indicated.

Limitations in the Use of Counseling Interviews

The counselor is responsible for the welfare of some persons for whom the counseling interview is not appropriate. The types of cases for which it is or has been regarded by others as inappropriate will be discussed in the following paragraphs.

Motivation of the client. We cannot force a person to become a client. We cannot force him to talk of his feelings and to change his meanings whether they pertain to fear of a dentist or doctor, or to shame of exposing his body to the examination of a physician. We cannot revise by mandate feelings of inadequacy associated with the loss of a limb, or with a cardiac condition, with extremes in height or weight, or with distortions about sexual behavior. We cannot alter an individual's feelings that lead to refusal to participate in physical education or social activities, by ordering him to change these feelings.

In an institution that has developed a counseling program built on understanding and respect for its students or other clients, they will come voluntarily seeking help. A counselor usually will not hesitate to take the initiative to bring the client to his office. The person assigned the responsibility for health counseling (a general counselor working in all problem areas or a specialist in the health area) may learn of a student's need from any of the following sources: written or oral reports from the physician, nurse, coach, teachers; parents; observations of his own; references to the student by other clients during interviews with them. Examples of these will be listed.

Written or oral reports from members of the staff. The physician informs the health counselor that a student resists necessary medical attention. The teacher notifies the counselor that a student bursts into tears when called on in class. The physical education instructor reports that the student on restricted activity program must be almost physically restrained from participating in the unlimited program. The dietician tells of a very obese girl who causes a commotion, attracting the attention of her classmates by eating two lunches and three desserts.

References to a student by other clients. A high-school student, discussing his own problem, refers to "that strange kid" in the class. This may be a function of the client's own "strangeness," but when repeated by others or corroborated by the counselor's observations, it deserves attention. A college student comes to talk about his morose roommate, a veteran who lost his hand in combat and who now avoids all social contacts except those involved in going to class, the cafeteria, and occasionally a theater.

Conversation with parents. One mother tells of her boy's nausea every Friday. The counselor discovers that Friday is oral-report day in his English class. Another mother states that her 5′10″ daughter has developed poor posture to look short enough to get dates, and asks for help.

Observations of the counselor. The counselor does not live in his office even if he is a full-time nonteaching counselor. As he walks in the corridor or visits in a class, he sees the fat child waddling along, the pallor of the seemingly undernourished child, the withdrawn, defensive behavior of the hard-of-hearing girl, and the hyperaggressive, overcompensating behavior of the undersized boy.

These are the students who have not come voluntarily to the counselor. For one or more reasons, discussed in the section on the unmotivated person, they are not moved to seek the assistance of the counselor. The counselor attempts to validate the clues and if they are confirmed, he invites the student to his office. In doing this, he knows that it may be of no value in producing change in the client. He recognizes, however, that it will provide him with an opportunity for observation; that it will establish the fact that the student is or is not ready to participate in counseling interviews; that it may indicate the need for informing other specialists of the student's symptoms; that it will demonstrate to the student that there is a person who accepts him as he is and is interested in helping him now or at such time as he, the client, desires help.

Let us see how the counselor handles the early stages of the interview with the unmotivated individual. For this purpose, we shall assume that Jim Doe does not come voluntarily to the counselor. In fact, the counselor learns through another teacher about this boy whose attitudes toward health, and toward men and women, interfere with his development.

Jim's English teacher, a man sensitive to the feelings of people, sends the counselor the following anecdotal report:

> Today at the beginning of class I asked James Doe to see me after class. Tears welled to his eyes. During class he seemed to be off in the distance. When I asked him after class if something was bothering him, he answered, "I hate this terrible acne."
>
> James tends to avoid the company of others. This seems to be happening more each day. He was never very sociable but now he is less so than earlier this semester.
>
> His behavior toward me is strange. Sometimes it seems as if he is afraid of me.

The counselor examined Jim's health record which was negative except for the acne. He spoke with Jim's teachers and learned that they had noticed his asocial tendencies. The counselor discussed Jim further with the English teacher and the two agreed that the counselor should ask Jim to come for an interview.

Jim stands at the doorway, his face tense and pale.

Counselor (warmly): Won't you come in, Jim, and have a seat.

Jim (hesitantly): Yes.

Counselor (slowly and softly): I'm very glad you were able to come today. Let me introduce myself. I'm called the counselor, and my job is to help students in any way I can. Some students come here to talk about making friends, some come to talk about taking care of their teeth, and some about gaining weight. I thought you might like to know about this.

Jim: I didn't know about this. Thank you.

Counselor: I wonder if I can be of any help to you.

Jim (flustered, in a tight voice): I . . . I don't know . . . I can't think of anything.

Counselor: You don't have to hurry, Jim. I've set aside twenty minutes for you. This is your time to use as you like. Maybe you want to just sit and think about it. You don't have to talk.

Maybe Jim will talk. If he does and if he evinces interest in this kind of help, the counselor will use the counseling interview. That will be his method of helping Jim achieve the changes in his meanings that will bring them closer to reality and that will enable him to satisfy his needs and will thus produce healthier living.

Maybe he will not be interested in counseling. In that event, the counselor cannot help him now by means of the interview. The counseling interview is inappropriate for the client who does not want counseling. It sometimes happens that a client who rejects the offer of counseling at a first interview like this returns voluntarily at a later date. The counselor who respects the right of the individual to accept or reject aid, who neither intimidates nor bribes to win him as a client, lays the groundwork for successful counseling. This occurs when the individual feels the need and returns as a motivated client to one who has respected him.

Some counselor will go one step farther with the unmotivated client than in the counseling described in the preceding paragraphs. He will introduce the problem area as he knows it in terms of Jim's symptoms. For example, he will ask Jim if he has friends; if he would like his help in gaining friends; if he would like help in dealing with the acne. Some positive step, in addition to that of introducing Jim to the counseling service available to him, can serve as a motivator. There is the danger, however, that it will open up an area which Jim is not yet prepared to face, and that this threat to Jim will endanger the possibility of his seeking aid from the counselor in the future, if and when he should desire help. Unfortunately, there is no rule of thumb method of determining when it is safe to open up the problem area with the unmotivated client and when it is not. The counselor must be able to sense the client's readiness, in terms of his seeming acceptance of the interview, his emotional state as evidenced by his posture, muscular tension in face and hands, and his apparent interest in continuing the relationship.

Qualities of the counselor. The health counselor who questions his ability to conduct counseling interviews will favor the case-work approach. This is a wholesome reaction for those persons who lack the qualities described in Chapter IV but who happen to have the responsibility for counseling. This is an unfortunate reaction when counselors avoid use of counseling interviews on the ground that they are inexperienced with it.

A counselor will find it desirable to experience counseling first under supervision, either the supervision of an instructor in a field-work course in counseling, or that of a department head on the job. Even after this educational experience, some counselors still feel unequipped for independent activity. The fact is that in counseling, as in many other fields, like teaching, medical work, coaching, and pastoral work, the young worker must accomplish much of his learning on the job. The counselor's first clients cannot have a polished counselor. This is an inevitable phenomenon in a society of mortal beings where new young workers must prepare to fill the places of those who die and retire. The young counselor who postpones interviewing activity because he is unequipped and uses case-work methods in its place will never learn to interview and deprives himself and his clients of the most effective instrument in helping individuals with their adjustment problems. He may also be operating on the false premise that errors in case-work methods and in manipulating the individual's environment are less harmful than errors in counseling.

The person with training in counseling, who has warm feelings for people, who can accept the values of others even when they disagree with his own, and who is sensitive to their feelings, can safely undertake counseling. It is far better that such people, aware of their limitations, perform the counseling functions consciously and officially, than that persons who advise, urge, moralize, or cajole perform these functions officially or unofficially. Unfortunately, they are being so performed in schools, colleges, and various other institutions throughout the country.

Time available. The type of counseling interview described in this book is frequently labeled as impracticable in institutions like the public schools. "There is not enough time to allow the client to go on talking about his problems. You have got to get to the point quickly, and the only way to do this is to see that the interview moves along quickly to a solution. This means that you have to tell him how to handle his problem." If this attitude were justified, then the counselor would collect and analyze data about an individual and present the facts to him, with or without the counselor's advice. This presupposes that providing an individual with facts will change his attitudes toward amputation, acne, size, limited activity, fear of death, tuberculosis. The nailbiter does not stop biting when she is told that she is biting because her height makes her tense and self-conscious. The meaning she has attached to height is not altered by these facts; and it is the meaning that shapes behavior. Surely, the enuretic (bed wetting) client does not terminate his annoying behavior when he is told that his enuresis is due to the fact that he senses that his mother rejects him.

The choice of the busy health counselor in working with individuals with problems—aside from the preventive aspects of the health program—is between an ineffective "quickie" information-giving or counselor-centered interview that achieves little or no change, and the admittedly more time-consuming interview that achieves change in meanings.

We are aware that counseling of this kind—utilizing the interview or the case-work approach—cannot be provided in many institutions. The staff members assigned to counseling responsibilities are so burdened with other duties that they cannot function in the manner described in this book. Funds are not made available for additional staff members, for persons who are adequately trained for this work. Administrators in some institutions are not genuinely in favor of such a "frill" as counseling and, at best, give only lip service to it. Whatever the reason for inadequate staff in the counseling area, let us not delude ourselves into believing that the quick counselor-dominated conversation between a harried counselor loaded with many clerical tasks and a disinterested client constitutes counseling.

Time is a limiting factor in the practice of good counseling wherever adequate counseling service is not provided. This applies as much to case-work methods as to the counseling interview.

Ability of the client. It is generally assumed that client-centered counseling demands average verbal ability, and that the prognosis is very poor with persons who have insufficient intelligence to cope with life situations independently. This would suggest that the case-work method of doing something to and for the client is essential for feeble-minded persons. Because this represents the thinking of many people working in this field it is a safe guide for the present.

The data of several studies suggest that this belief may not be a valid one. Scientists studying mental ability, as measured by intelligence tests, have recognized the role of environment. The conclusions of most such people may be summed up in the words of Super:[1]

> . . . whereas both nature and nurture play a part in the development of intelligence, mental ability as indicated by the intelligence quotient is relatively constant from the time a child enters elementary school until late adulthood. It is true that the obtained I.Q. will vary some after the age of six, but this is generally more a function of the tests, which

[1] Donald E. Super, *Appraising Vocational Fitness,* New York: Harper and Bros., 1949; p. 87.

are often not strictly comparable at different age levels and which are in any case subject to errors of measurement, than of the individual. Some changes which are too great to be explained by these causes are the result of emotional conditions which invalidate the score of one test, or of organic changes resulting from disease or injury. That there are other changes, not explained by any of these factors and attributable to changes in the environment which modify the functioning intelligence, has not been demonstrated to the satisfaction of all competent judges with persons of elementary school age or older."

A number of studies place much greater stress on the influence of the environment on the intellectual functioning of the individual. The work of Warner[2] and his associates, the controversial study of Schmidt,[3] and the research of Pasamanack[4] on intelligence of Negro infants suggest that persons who are underprivileged, who are made to feel unwanted, who, in other words, develop self-concepts associated with unworthiness and unacceptance, are inefficient in their learning. Since intelligence tests presuppose approximately equal opportunity to learn, these persons are at a disadvantage.

If distorted meanings create the conditions for what we call mental retardation, then it would appear that counseling which changes meanings of the self may alter the mental-ability status. At least, such counseling would create the condition by which the individual could learn without disadvantage. Research is necessary to determine whether a client-centered counseling relationship may not be actually indicated with such persons.

Deficient verbal ability is frequently raised as an insuper-

[2] W. Lloyd Warner, Robert J. Havinghurst, and Martin B. Loeb, *Who Shall Be Educated?* New York: Harper and Bros., 1944.

[3] Bernardine G. Schmidt, "Changes in Personal, Social and Intellectual Behavior of Children Originally Classified as Feebleminded," *Psychological Monograph* 60 (1946) No. 5. See also the adverse critique by S. A. Kirk and a reply by Schmidt in *Psychological Bulletin,* 45, 321-343 (1948).

[4] Benjamin Pasamanack, "A Comparative Study of the Behavioral Development of Negro Infants," *Journal of Genetic Psychology,* 69, 3-44 (1946).

able barrier to effective use of the counseling interview with the mentally retarded. Dorfman[5] reports on a successful counseling relationship with a boy who rarely verbalized. This boy was not mentally deficient, but he showed no inclination to communicate verbally. Apparently, changes in meaning can occur as a result of a counseling relationship in which the counselor *can accept* the silence of the client.

The Unmotivated Person

Who is the person who does not come voluntarily for counseling, but deserves the attention of the counselor?

Sometimes he is a student in high school, college, or nursing school, or a member of the general community who simply does not know that counseling facilities are available to him. In this case, he would be a motivated client if he were properly oriented.

Sometimes he knows of the counseling service, but is repelled by the seeming lack of warmth and interest on the part of the counselors, or a lack of trust in their ethical practices. The quality of relationship a counselor develops soon becomes known, and it affects the desire of students to utilize it. The need for self-aggrandizement of some persons serving as counselors sometimes leads them to discuss the spectacular content of an intimate counseling interview. This violation of professional trust can cause grave harm to the counseling program of the institution.

The act of discussing with a stranger (the counselor) one's personal problems requires a great deal of strength from persons who are not accustomed to expose their feelings. The pain created by their problem must outweigh the pain of such a release. When an individual has ambivalent feelings, that is, attraction toward and replusion from something like counseling, the stronger feeling determines behavior. There may be vacillation and indecision, but when the stronger emotion

[5] Elaine Dorfman, "Play Therapy," chapter 6 in Carl R. Rogers' *Client-Centered Therapy*, New York: Houghton-Mifflin, 1951, p. 244-247.

is antagonistic to counseling, the individual is then unmotivated for counseling.

Some persons do not seek counseling because the threat of being "adjusted" is greater than the pain of maladjustment. Here is a paraplegic who sits sullenly in his wheel chair. Perhaps his self-concept is that of a worthless, unattractive person. He is terrified by the thoughts he has of himself and will do anything to avoid reminders of what he represents for himself. When people stare at him, pity him, or seek to aid him, they reinforce these feelings. Therefore, he seeks to avoid being placed in situations that provoke such reminders. This requires isolation and isolation excludes counseling.

The maladjusted person uses one or more of a variety of ineffective adjustive mechanisms, usually known as defense mechanisms, to cope with his situation. The individual who comes for counseling voluntarily has not been content with the manner in which his defenses have handled the situation for him.

Many of the persons whom we classify as maladjusted and unmotivated for counseling have found means of coping with their situations. For example, let us return to our paraplegic. Let us say that when his mother asks him why he does not accept invitations to visit friends he replies that these friends are too frivolous. Their interests are not serious like his, he says, for he has had experiences that are beyond them. He wants to go to their houses, fears going, and now gives a socially acceptable reason for refusing to go. This mechanism is known as rationalization. The rationalization is a defense against criticism. It is a defense that maintains the self in that it protects the paraplegic from experiences which to him signify the inadequacies of his self. It is a defense that even enhances the self, for the paraplegic is attributing to himself certain esteemed qualities. But he does this at a cost to himself of social participation. We observers classify him as maladjusted and arrange an interview with him because we believe that his adjustment is not a healthful one. When he tells us during the interview what he has told his mother, we accept this as we accept his other feelings in our attempt to create the relationship that will lead him to reorganize his perceptions. If he continues with us, he will find less need for defense by rationalization. He will accept his paraplegia as we accept it. He will come to see himself more clearly, recognizing his worthiness and attractiveness. He will then have the courage to exchange social participation, which enhances, for rationalization, which enhances but also isolates.

If he cannot accept the counseling relationship, then he can be aided, if at all, through the case-work approach.

Adjustment mechanisms such as rationalization are not unique to maladjusted persons. All of us utilize one or more of these. We learn during childhood that certain reasons for staying out of school, such as feeling sick, are acceptable, whereas others, like fear of a scheduled examination, are not acceptable, even if they are the honest ones. We learn that our parents are more tolerant of our poor performance in school if we blame the teacher or distractions in the classroom. We learn these so well that they become part of our everyday behavior. When we are in college we rationalize to make palatable to ourselves a behavior that we have come to regard as being undesirable. For example, being unprepared for an examination has negative meaning to the college student. Going to a movie before an examination when one is unprepared is acceptable only when one can satisfy oneself that "it isn't good to study the night before an exam. You should relax. That's what psychologists say."

While these mechanisms are employed by all of us, maladjusted persons use them to a degree that makes these persons qualitatively different from the normal in behavior. The counselor who is familiar with this variety of adjustive behavior is better equipped to understand the development of meanings in an individual.[6]

[6] For detailed description of these mechanisms see Laurance F. Shaffer, *Psychology of Adjustment,* New York: Houghton-Mifflin, 1936, Part II, pp. 143-280.

STUDYING THE INDIVIDUAL

The counselor is seeking to help Jim, a student who appears to need help. As we have seen, the English teacher has sent the counselor an *anecdotal record.* This has led him to search for further facts that will explain Jim's asocial behavior and his strong feelings about acne, and that will lead to action to produce wholesome changes. The anecdotal record is a brief description of an episode or occurrence in the life of a student, prepared by the observer. Cumulative anecdotes provide a picture of the student's conduct and personality and a record of his development. In our large schools and for the busy health counselor, perusal of such records will bring to light students in need of one or another health service. Discovery by this means of a counseling or other need can spare the student undue misery and possibly avoid a more serious problem.

The counselor examines the *cumulative record,* a term which one writer[7] applies "to all records that make provision for the accumulation of significant and comprehensive information about an individual pupil over a period of years." This would include the anecdotal records or at least information transcribed from them to a cumulative record form. It also includes subjects taken, grades, psychological test results, information about home and family, about hobbies and extracurricular activities, about attendance and discipline. Some cumulative records indicate the nature of any health condition that would affect any aspect of adjustment of the individual, whether scholastic, social, or vocational. The counselor studying Jim would search for evidence in the cumulative record of changes in general performance in school, for information on his attendance, and for reactions of teachers that may be noted on it. This record provides a longitudinal picture of Jim during the years of his school attendance, and

[7] Arthur E. Traxler, *Techniques of Guidance,* New York: Harper and Bros., 1945; p. 215.

careful analysis reveals inconsistencies or sharp deviations.

He checks on Jim's health with the school physician or nurse who will discuss with him any significant medical findings.

He wants to have the benefit of the observations of Jim's *teachers*. He speaks with Jim's current teachers and with those from previous years, if they are available.

The counselor has taken this information, examined it carefully and decided that the English teacher's observations are confirmed. He asks Jim to come to his office. The *interview* provides the counselor with further information, for it discloses Jim's fear of this relationship and his rejection of further interviews.

The counselor knows that he must rely on forces external to Jim to bring about changes in meanings. Unfortunately, he does not possess the knowledge of the boy's background that we have. He seeks to accumulate as much information as will provide a sound basis for manipulating Jim and his environment. He is searching for Jim's distorted meanings. He arranges with one or two teachers to sit in the classroom for *personal observation* of Jim. He is prepared to look for specific types of behavior. Does Jim come in by himself? Does he talk with his neighbors before class starts? Does he pick on his acne scabs when he thinks he is unnoticed? What are his reactions to class activity? Does he daydream?

The counselor may also arrange to talk with one or both of Jim's parents. He will talk with them to learn more about Jim by knowing something about the outlook of his parents. Perhaps he will sense the mother's frustration and guilt about her boy's acne and her attitude toward health. He will be careful to conduct this interview in such a way that any future relationship with Jim will not be impaired. He will not want the parents to feel shame in discussing Jim and especially not to feel the need to put further pressure on Jim. This is not easy to avoid. One investigation[8] suggests that when

[8] B. Merrill, "A Measurement of Mother Child Interaction," *Journal of Abnormal and Social Psychology*, 41, p. 49 (1946).

parents are informed that their children have not worked up to capacity, they will try to drive the children all the more. The fact that a counselor discusses a child with his parent has come to mean that the child's performance or behavior is unsatisfactory. The counselor will not use the interview to blame, condemn, or preach. He knows he cannot change their meanings of health or morality, or their feelings toward Jim except by counseling them as motivated clients, and the interview with the parents is not for that purpose. He will use it to learn more about Jim's parents and thus be better prepared to help Jim. If in the process the parents gain some insight into their attitudes toward their son, all the better.

The counselor has collected data from these many sources, and now prepares a *case study*. He does this partly to have a comprehensive, well-organized record available to all of the counseling team members; and partly as a discipline that enables him to recognize the dynamics in Jim's behavior and the trends in his development. The case study has been described by Strang[9] as "a synthesis and interpretation of information about a person and his relationship to his environment, collected by means of many technics. . . . At its best, it is a personality picture that becomes clearer and more lifelike as each new item is added. . . . To accomplish these ends requires psychological insight and critical thinking based on the best available data viewed as a whole. The case study helps the counselor understand the nature and causes of an individual's behavior, personality trends, and difficulties in adjustment."

The counselor cannot learn the meanings that Jim has acquired for his self, his parents, health, and acne through the counseling interview, for Jim, as we discuss him now, is not a motivated client. He can do the next best thing: infer Jim's meanings from his behavior.

The *case conference* is a further means of studying the

[9] Ruth Strang, *Counseling Technics in College and Secondary School,* New York: Harper and Bros., 1949, p. 207.

individual. It is described in the next section because of its great value in mobilizing the members of a faculty.

Manipulating the Environment

The *case conference* is an exceedingly valuable instrument of the counselor. It is used by a variety of professional workers, all of them aware of the advantages of team work in the jobs of human relations.

The counselor arranges a meeting of those persons on the staff who are familiar with the case and those who may be called on to help. The student's current teachers will be invited and perhaps some from previous years. Depending on the nature of the problem, the school physician, school psychologist, visiting teacher, nurse, and representatives of agencies familiar with the case or possibly helpful in working out a plan of action will also be invited. The counselor will make a brief statement on the case. In a conference dealing with the unmotivated Jim, he might start by asking the English teacher to report on his experiences with Jim. The counselor will then ask for contributions from others present who are familiar with the case. When the situation is understood, the counselor will lead a discussion exploring causative factors and possible means of aiding the individual involved.

Many gains come from the case conference. 1. The members leave with a design for action, tentative as it may be. 2. They are sensitized to the client's need for understanding and help; from then on he is not just a member of a class; he is one who deserves special attention. 3. Teachers are sensitized to the needs of all students for something more than just the three R's and their high school equivalents. 4. They develop from it respect for the aims of counseling and greater respect for those assigned the counseling responsibilities in the institution. 5. They feel that they have been consulted in a counseling problem and now assume some responsibility for a share of the counseling work. 6. They come to see "the relationship of physical, intellectual, social, and emotional factors."[10]

Many agencies and institutions that have a counseling service, including some schools, have a scheduled case conference each week, or at some other time interval. Those responsible for counseling attend regularly, and other persons are invited in so far as they are involved or can be helpful in the case scheduled for discussion.

What are the specific case-work techniques of the counselor in producing changed meanings in the client? Before seeking an answer to this question, let us consider the nature of the client. Despite the great variety of symptoms found among them, a few threads run through so many of the cases that these may be regarded as typical. They are typical whether the client is a tall stoop-shouldered girl, or an arrested tuberculosis case, an amputee, or an adolescent disturbed by budding feelings of sex. The self-concept is that of a threatened person, and the individual feels inadequate, unsuccessful, or unattractive. These feelings may appear to be limited to only one province of activity, such as academic performance, or social activities, or heterosexual relations, or it may appear to be generalized to all activities. The inadequacy may be reflected in the client's inability to accept his own values, which are consistent with his own needs, as against the dominating values of authoritarian influences in his life. Jim may feel like eating a hot dog at a ball game, as his classmates are doing, and eating it will satisfy his need to be like them as well as his gustatory needs! But the value of eating the hot dog that he now experiences is dominated by the negative value he has acquired from his mother. From her, he has learned that such food is bad.

To counter these meanings the individual has attached to himself, to give him strength to see his positive as well as negative qualities, the counselor attempts to *promote close*

[10] Ruth Strang, *Counseling Technics in College and Secondary School,* New York: Harper and Bros., 1949, p. 211.

relations between the individual and teachers and other students. The teachers who attended the case conference will make special effort to improve their relationship with him. They will try to greet him each day without making this obvious; they will show interest in him as he works at his desk; they will get him involved in class activity, such as committee work.

The counselor will seek *to promote successful experiences to establish a sense of worth.* Again, he must depend largely on the student's teachers, and on faculty advisors to extracurricular activities, if the student is engaged in them. Imaginative teachers have searched patiently in the records of a child for evidence of some skill that would elevate him above mediocrity in his own eyes. Some have taken mediocrity itself and candy-coated it to light a spark of self-respect or worthiness and adequacy in the child. The story has been told [11] of the teacher who took a simple drawing by a highly withdrawn adolescent with mediocre ability in art, as in all his other performance, framed it attractively and posted it on the school's bulletin board. A large notice beneath it described it as first winner of the "Picture of the Week" award. The boy now gained a new importance for students and faculty, and the unexpected success gave new self-meanings to him. What is of perhaps the greatest significance is the fact that members of the faculty, who were involved in the study of the boy and in implementing the plan of action, showed an increased interest in him which he felt.

Another example of the creative efforts of a teacher is reported by Bullis and O'Malley:[12]

[11] H. Edmund Bullis, in address at the 1951 Convention of the Council on Guidance and Personal Association.

[12] H. Edmund Bullis, and Emily E. O'Malley, *Human Relations in the Classroom,* Wilmington: The Delaware State Society for Mental Hygiene, 1948. Among the sample lesson plans in this book are: "How Personality Traits Develop," "How Emotions Affect Us Physically," "Public Enemies of Good Relations," "Overcoming Personal Handicaps," "That Inferiority Feeling," "Why Daydream, Why Relax." A second volume has been published: H. Edmund Bullis, *Human Relations in the Classroom, Course II,* Wilmington: The Delaware Society for Mental Hygiene, 1948.

One of the finest examples I know of a teacher's ingenuity in helping a shy child took place in Toronto, Canada. In one of the classes where we were studying shy children some nine years ago, the teacher had one boy whom she could not get to speak loud enough in class to be heard by the rest of the children. For weeks she tried to give the shy, timid youngster, David, more confidence. She endeavored to learn if there were anything he could do a little better than the rest of the children. This was difficult, for David seemed to be an average boy in every way, other than for his extreme timidity. One noon when she was approaching the school, she noticed him riding his bike on the sidewalk just in front of her. He would ride very slowly for a foot or two more. When the teacher came up to him, she said, "Dave, you certainly can ride a bike slowly, can't you?" She could barely hear his quiet, "Yes, Ma'am."

As she proceeded to the school, she had an idea. That afternoon she put it into execution. She borrowed a pail of whitewash from the janitor; then she had the boys in her class line out, in the back yard of the school, a series of parallel lines, about ten feet apart, extending from fence to fence. The next day in school she invited all children who had bikes to bring them to school that afternoon, and the first "slow-riding bicycle race" in history was put on. The rules were simple. All the children started from one fence and had to stay within the space between the whitewashed lines allotted them. Touching the ground with the feet or running over the line disqualified the offender. David won the race with no trouble and became the "slow-riding bicycle champion" of his class.

The following day the contest was open to the students in the higher classes in the school and again he won easily. He became the "slow-riding bicycle champion" of the school. Much interest was aroused, and other schools in that part of Toronto were challenged, with the result that David became the "slow-riding bicycle champion" in that area of Toronto.

While these contests were going on, all of the children in his class and—for that matter—in his school, started looking on David as a hero, for he was the only champion of which their school could boast. The other boys and girls wanted him to participate in all of their school affairs and made a great fuss over him. As the weeks went by, his personality changed decidedly. The fact that he was given recognition and was sought out so much by other children changed his entire outlook on life. Without realizing it, he was talking above a whisper in class when called on, and gradually his shy and timid mannerisms disappeared almost entirely. David could never become an extrovert, but he did—due to the integrity of his teacher—gain self-confidence to the point that he became one of the most popular boys in his class.

An *interview with a parent* may be conducted now not for informational purposes as before, but to achieve parental understanding of the child's needs. These may be beyond the power of a parent to satisfy, as, for example, the child's need for love from a rejecting parent. But a parent may wish to help in dealing with personal inadequacies which she recognizes as affecting her child. In this case, the counselor informs the parent of professional services in the community.

The counselor and the faculty seek to instill in the student a sense of belonging, *of being part of a group*. They attempt to achieve this by use of a variety of *group activities* discussed next. The group activities have still another important role to the health counselor; they *provide information about health and physiological functioning to offset the ignorance and misinformation that contribute to the making of health problems.*

Group Activities

This section embraces the discussion activities in health education classes, in home-room and subject classes, in the special adjustment class, the human relations class, and in extracurricular activities that focus on the attitudes and problems of the students. Classes of this kind, so different from the traditional class, are concerned with the problems of their members rather than with the content of a book. This also applies to activities with similar focus and conducted in community agencies, settlement houses, churches, young people's organizations, hospitals, and other institutions.

Let us study a session of this kind. Jim is a member of the class in health education. The teacher has described the problem of a boy who had had infantile paralysis and now walked with a slight limp. The boy thought he should not go to parties. The teacher asked the students what they thought.

Mary: Well, I think he should. Even if he can't dance, he can have fun.

Bill: Even with a limp he can dance. And what's the difference if he can't dance?

Joe: He's as good as anyone else. What if he does have a limp?

George: But maybe people will stare and no one likes people staring at you.

Betty (sharply): Let them stare, if they're stupid. I have a big birth mark on my thigh right here above my knee, but it doesn't keep me from going swimming. (Several boys titter.) Why don't you boys grow up?

Celia: A lot of us don't have everything the way we want it, but it doesn't mean we won't have fun.

Lewis: Look at this wart (points to a wart near his chin). I don't like it, but so what? If anyone doesn't like me because of that, I don't want to know that person.

Harold: And here I thought I was the only one who felt funny about being different. I never used to like anyone to see I was lacking a finger.

And so it goes on, young people projecting their own meanings and values into the discussion, and gaining insight into their own problems. This is learning that remains long after a final exam! Jim has not participated, but he is experiencing it. Perhaps Harold has expressed Jim's feelings that he, too, thought he was the only one. Perhaps he, too, will find the courage in this permissive classroom atmosphere to speak up and thus to speed up the process of change. Perhaps he will begin to share the "belongingness" that comes from feeling part of a group of this kind. Here he has a chance to feel accepted, liked, secure. Just as he is learning that others with physical defects accept them and do not withdraw into a shell, so he may learn that other students have ambivalent feelings toward their parents. He may learn, too, that others seek help from a counselor. Participation in such a group frequently makes a motivated client out of an unmotivated person.

The benefits of such dynamic group processes are not limited to persons who are in need of help. Discussions of this type constitute a mental hygiene program designed to eliminate distorted meanings and to prevent the incidence of distorted behavior like that of Jim's. The catharsis that comes from release of feelings is one specific value; the knowledge that one's peers have similar problems removes the impression that one's problems are unique and unmentionable and serves to lend support to the individual; finally, it has its therapeutic value in its ability to change meanings, for example, that acne is just acne, and that like a wart or a limp, it is shared by others, it is not uncommon, and it does not lead to unattractiveness or unworthiness.

A good counseling program in health, as in other areas, includes both individual and group counseling. The group technique is more economical in time and staff. It supplements individual counseling, often serving as a "recruiting ground" for the counselor, helping to detect those who need help, and helping to motivate the unmotivated. Finally, the unmotivated client has access to the group activity, especially when it is one of the regular classes.

There is much that teachers and health workers in America have done to help our people develop concepts of their selves and to choose values that are more in accord with the reality of their needs. The sum of this creative effort could not be recorded in one volume even if all of it were known.

Not all efforts of the counselor will be fruitful. Conditions like the following limit the counselor's achievement; undernourishment due to low family income; marital discord of parents; resistance of many employers to the hiring of handicapped workers; social mores that conflict sharply with physiological need. The counselor recognizes that many of these frustrating conditions require more than counseling. The social conditions that produced them need revaluation and correction. As citizen, the counselor may wish to promote such action. As counselor, he utilizes the counseling interview and the case-work approach to help individuals so far as these limitations permit.

Bibliography

Arbuckle, Dugald S., *Teacher Counseling,* Cambridge: Addison-Wesley Press, 1950, chapters 5 and 6.

Bingham, Walter V. D., and Bruce V. Moore, *How to Interview,* New York: Harper and Bros., 1941, chapter 11.

Bullis, H. Edmund, *Human Relations in the Classroom, Course II,* Wilmington: The Delaware Society for Mental Hygiene, 1948.

Bullis, H. Edmund, and Emily E. O'Malley, *Human Relations in the Classroom, Course I,* Wilmington: The Delaware State Society for Mental Hygiene, 1947.

Cantor, Nathaniel, *The Dynamics of Learning,* Buffalo: Foster and Stewart Publishing Corp., 1946. A significant and challenging book on new goals and new methods in education.

Hahn, Milton E., and Melcolm S. MacLean, *General Clinical Counseling,* New York: McGraw-Hill, 1950, chapters 5 and 6.

Hoppock, Robert, *Group Guidance,* New York: McGraw-Hill, 1949.

Robinson, Francis P., *Principles and Procedures in Student Counseling,* New York: Harper and Bros., 1950, chapter 11.

Rogers, Carl R., *Client-Centered Therapy,* New York: Houghton Mifflin, 1951. See chapters 7, 8, and 9.

Slavson, S. R., *An Introduction to Group Therapy,* New York: Commonwealth Fund, 1943.

Snygg, Donald, and Arthur W. Combs, *Individual Behavior, A*

New Frame of Reference for Psychology, New York: Harper and Bros., 1949, chapter 13.

Strang, Ruth, *Counseling Technics in College and Secondary School,* New York: Harper and Bros., 1949.

Wiles, Kimball, *Supervision for Better Schools,* New York: Prentice-Hall, 1950. The application of a philosophy like ours to the problems of leadership, staff morale, improvement of staff meetings, coordination of staff activities.

Chapter VIII

A PHYSICIAN LOOKS AT HEALTH COUNSELING

The Medical Philosophy of Counseling

Just as there must be a philosophy underlying counseling, if it is to contribute to the growth of the counselee, so must there be a philosophy underlying the health aspects of this field, a philosophy which to the modern physician or other health specialist has at least two fundamental principles.

The first principle assumes that health is a *positive force* in life, that we must approach health with the realization that it is one of our most valuable assets. As so aptly phrased in the constitution of the World Health Organization, "Health is a state of complete physical, mental, and social well-being and not merely the absence of disease and infirmity." The negative approach which says in effect, "You must develop good health habits or you will get tuberculosis, or rheumatic fever, or a communicable disease" creates an atmosphere of constant threat from hostile forces, which in itself is not conducive to health. The slogan, "It's wonderful to know you're healthy," recognizes the value of the positive concept.

This view of health does not ignore the possible results of poor health habits. A teen-ager who pushes sleep into the background because, "I don't want to miss any fun," and diets so that she can wear a size 12 dress may seriously injure herself. She may find herself in a hospital where several months of bed rest will be necessary to arrest a minimal tuberculosis lesion in her lung. Illnesses do exist in the world and refusal to acknowledge their existence does not automatically banish them. The wise mother does not tell her small daughter that the stove isn't hot. She will help her child understand what fire is, and the penalty for playing with it, but she will not make the presence of the stove in the kitchen a dominating fear in the life of her child. Knowledge of disease produces a gnawing fear that detracts constantly from one's ability to enjoy life, lest one catch a cold, or receive an injury that might develop into cancer, only in one who has a negative concept of health. St. Augustine, in the fifth century, observing the evil in the world resulting from immorality, might have said, "Don't enter into the pursuits of life that bring physical enjoyment or you will suffer." Instead he uttered words that stated a profound truth and became famous, "Love God and do as you please!" The person who thinks of health in such terms says in effect, "Love health; live according to physical, mental, and social rules for health, letting them become an integral part of your daily habits, and you will find yourself enjoying life to the full."

Consider the attitude of the man who purchases a new car. He is proud of its glistening surface and smooth performance. He dusts and washes it regularly. He drives more carefully, hoping to maintain its original finish. He checks frequently to see that there is water in the radiator, that the proper oil level is maintained, that the battery plates are covered with water, that the gasoline he uses is clean. He has an expert mechanic grease the car at regular intervals and look over such parts as steering wheel and brakes. He starts with a piece of machinery that is good both in appearance and function and he develops certain habits, follows certain patterns in the care of that machinery which will make him feel that his car will stay new as long as possible.

Similarly, the individual who recognizes health as one of the great assets in his life will develop in the achievement of his goals, whether mental or physical, habits of health, not because he constantly fears the penalties that may come from poor practices, but because he is intensely interested in keeping or improving his health status. The health counselor who can help a child or an adult arrive at this concept is a valuable member of a health team.

The second principle on which the physician bases his philosophy of the health aspects of good counseling is that *maturity in matters of health means the acceptance by the individual of responsibility for his own health.* This principle may be challenged. Should a growing child be allowed to assume responsibility for his own health to an increasing degree? Many physicians would question such a statement, saying that the child does not realize the serious consequences of failure to follow health rules, that the family doctor, in times of illness, and the parents, in times of health, should be very directive in the health approach and establish certain definite rules which the child must follow.

The parents themselves frequently hesitate to agree with such a principle, being fearful that their children will become ill. Mary's mother had studied enough psychology to be convinced that her daughter needed to develop independence of thought and action. She boasted about Mary's color sense at the age of ten, and about her ability to decide which dress and hair ribbon she would wear to school. Now that Mary is in high school, her mother is happy to see signs of her maturing in the way she makes her own decisions regarding her hours for home work, her extracurricular activities, or her choice of boy friends. She trusts Mary in allowing her to make some decisions because she feels that she has done what she could since Mary's infancy to lay the basis for sound judgment and wise action. She realizes that Mary is not yet an adult either physically or emotionally. She is there to guide her daughter toward wise choices, but she follows a general policy of keeping in the background. Likewise, since

Mary's preschool days, her mother has gradually taught her good health habits, explaining the health facts behind the practices, as far as Mary could understand them, and adding to those facts as Mary grew older. However, should she trust Mary's judgment on questions of health? "No, that would be foolish," she says. "If Mary should go to a football game on a cold November day with only a light coat, it might mean pneumonia!" So her mother continues to remind Mary that she should wear rubbers, or take an umbrella, or that she must get more sleep, or eat more fresh fruits and vegetables. Mary is a well-balanced, clear-thinking high-school student, one who will appreciate the opportunity to make her own decisions on health matters. Her mother can still be in the background until Mary becomes fully mature, but she should not deprive Mary of the chance for a gradual growth toward maturity.

When an individual has a positive concept of health, and has learned to be self-directive in health matters, he does not need counseling help except in times of crisis, and even then, he may be able to make the necessary emotional adjustments. He will utilize his health assets to the fullest extent. If disease or defect occurs, he will obtain scientific medical help, and will adjust to any change in his life that becomes necessary. But for the individual who is fearful, and who depends on parent, husband, wife, or friend when a decision must be made, illness will often result in tensions and maladjustment which he will be unable to cope with by himself. At such times, the physician recognizes the need for intelligent, trained persons to cooperate as a team in preventing illness or in dealing with the physical and emotional aspects of illness.

The Team-Work Approach to Health Counseling

Medicine today has grown to such an extent that no physician considers himself adequate to meet every situation. The best-qualified family doctor, the general practitioner, tries to keep abreast of scientific advances in all fields, but when his patient becomes acutely ill and the diagnosis is not clear, or when he needs surgery, the family doctor will turn to the specialist. In many parts of our country, the recognition that specialists are necessary has resulted in the formation of medical centers or group practice, where under one roof, a patient can be referred to an orthopedist, a surgeon, a dermatologist, gynecologist, pediatrician, obstetrician, or other specialist. He may also have laboratory tests done, or X-ray studies made. This all represents team work in the practice of medicine.

This approach is equally applicable to mental illness. For a number of years, such teams have made possible the improvements in state hospitals for mentally ill patients that have resulted in medical and psychiatric treatment instead of mere custodial care. The psychiatrist, psychiatric nurse, clinical psychologist, psychiatric social worker, hospital chaplain, physiotherapist, and occupational therapist have combined their efforts in the attempt to bring the patient back to contact with reality, to make him able to adjust to his family, and eventually to his job and his community. Now the significance of team work has reached into the area of private psychiatric practice. In Los Angeles, two psychiatrists have developed such a private-practice team over the last four years. In describing their procedure in the Journal of the American Medical Association, they state: "Meanwhile, the psychiatric team swings into full action. With the psychiatrist directing and supervising at crucial points, the patient utilizes the help of psychotherapists, psychologists, social workers, vocational counselors, teachers, and the leaders of group activities, as indicated in his particular case. . . . The successful operation of the team-work program requires that each worker be kept fully aware at all times that he is dealing with only one facet of the patient's problems and that he is, in the truest sense of the term, a member of the team. . . . A single person cannot do the job alone if the enormous and growing need for psychiatric help is to be met." [1]

These team members, however, have all had medical training in their special fields. In the minds of many health educators, classroom teachers, and guidance counselors is still arising this question, "When a student has an illness and is receiving medical care, will the physician in charge of diagnosis and treatment resent interference by someone whom he feels is not qualified to give advice about disease?" Before considering this question, it may be helpful to look at some contemporary facts. One such fact is that the horizons of the medical profession have broadened by the rapid advance through research in all branches of medicine, until the idea of a team to gain optimum results has been widely accepted. A second fact is the appalling lack of personnel as compared to the need. It is a recognized fact that the psychiatrists in the United States today represent a woefully inadequate number to deal with those patients who have been diagnosed as suffering from mental illness, those who are prepsychotic, and all those whose mental illness might be entirely prevented if problems causing tension and maladjustment could be dealt with before they produce serious conditions. The efforts not only of those who have adequate health background, such as health educators, but of every classroom teacher and parent can be enlisted to help solve those problems. Whether the individual needing help lacks attitudes and motivation for the establishment of good health habits in childhood or adolescent years, or whether he finds it difficult to adjust to a physical defect that will remain with him for life, the counselor who helps him becomes part of a team.

How then will a health-counseling team function? If we look at a school situation, we may find a typical team at work. A classroom teacher may refer a child who complains of feel-

[1] Esther Tietz, M.D., and Martin Grotjahn, M.D.: "Psychiatric Teamwork—An Integrated Therapy," *J.A.M.A.*, 145. No. 14, 1057 (1951).

ing ill to the school health office. If this happens during class, she may not be able to talk to the child at length, but since she knows that the doctor is in the building, she sends the child to him with a word of understanding and reassurance. The nurse greets the child, and, after learning some of his symptoms and taking his temperature and pulse rate, she goes with him into the doctor's office. The doctor may find definite illness and through the parents refer the child to medical specialists either as a private or as a clinic patient. In the school, the doctor depends on the nurse to work with him and with the child. The nurse, in turn, depends on the classroom teacher and, through nurse-teacher conferences, acquaints the teacher with the part she can play in helping the child to adjust to his illness as far as the classroom situation is concerned. This would refer to a situation where the illness did not necessitate the child's absence from school, or during the days after return to school. If the teacher has the personality, skill, and the knowledge for health counseling, the team as far as school personnel is concerned may be complete at this point. It may be necessary to enlarge the team to include the school guidance counselor, or the health educator, or someone outside of the school, such as a social worker. The child might be considered to be at the very heart of the team because of our concept of the nature of counseling. Members of the team are not doing something *to* the child. He is an active participant. He may accept help from experts but that help is not in the form of a prescription that starts with a command. If the counseling is wise and constructive, the help will be in the form of a permissive attitude and a sympathetic understanding that will enable the child to grow to the place where he can "write his own prescription" as to the best way to adjust to and develop in a given health situation. The child must be helped to grow to this place because it is he who will have to live with his illness or defect. The parent or teacher cannot be constantly at his side, directing his activity and his rest. As he learns with the help of counseling to meet his own problems, he will gradually mature beyond the need for further counseling.

The Physician Reviews the Qualifications of the Health Counselor

In considering the question as to whether or not the physician might resent participation on a health counseling team by a classroom teacher or other comparable person, the phrase "qualified to give advice" was used. The need for team work would appear to be acute. The progressive physician recognizes this fact, but he feels that every member of the team should meet at least two requirements or qualifications: He should be a good counselor and he should know the health facts regarding the particular problem concerned in any situation for which he does counseling.

The qualifications for a good counselor have been considered in an earlier chapter. The need of respect for and the liking of people is as important to the physician as it is to the classroom teacher or the professional counselor. It is interesting to note that in the opening chapter of a recent book on internal medicine, the suggestions given in our earlier chapter are almost paraphrased. In discussing the management of the patient the author states: "Tact, sympathy, and understanding are expected of the physician, for the patient is no mere collection of symptoms, signs, disordered functions, damaged organs, and disturbed emotions. He is human, fearful, and hopeful, seeking relief, help, and reassurance. To the physician, as to the anthropologist, nothing human is strange or repulsive. . . . The true physician has a Shakespearean breadth of interest in the wise and the foolish, the proud and the humble, the stoic hero and the whining rogue. He cares for people." [2] The ability to be permissive, to understand and to accept, is of utmost importance in helping the

[2] T. R. Harrison, *Principles of Internal Medicine,* Philadelphia: The Blakiston Co., 1950, p. 5.

person with a health problem. The physician, in his attempt to understand his patient and in his desire to have the patient understand himself, welcomes the help of any qualified person, for knowledge of the patient, not just of his symptoms, is necessary. "It is more important to know what kind of fellow has the germ, than to know what kind of germ has the fellow."[3]

The second requirement of a health counselor from a physician's view point is that the counselor should know the health facts concerning the problem. This is essential for a number of reasons. In the first place, knowledge of the facts will result in prompter referral when that is necessary. The student who comes to a teacher or counselor for help may be a sick person physically and emotionally. The ability to recognize the normal and to screen for possible illness or defect, together with the ability to help the student see the need for medical and psychiatric referral may mean an important step forward in the direction of the total adjustment of the student. This screening process cannot be based on good intentions or the mere desire to help. The classroom teacher who conducts Snellen tests in screening for children who may have defects of vision has been taught the significance of the test and the proper method of administering it. She does not know how to carry out an eye refraction test, how to examine eye grounds, or how to prescribe glasses, but she does know the facts necessary to do her part intelligently to assist in the preservation of eyesight.

Knowledge of facts will also enable the health counselor to help the student adjust to his illness while he is under the care of the physician, if the illness does not prevent his attendance at school. People who are ill, or who deviate from the normal, like to talk about their conditions. They want reassurance that the illness is not serious, that the defect is not too great, or too noticeable. The physician may spend

[3] Dr. Harry Wilmer, Palo Alto Clinic, California, in an address at the Annual Meeting of 1950 of the New York Tuberculosis and Health Association.

time during an office visit to explain the illness or defect, but the next day new worries may appear to the student. Then, he may turn to his teacher whom he likes and with whom he feels free to talk. If the teacher knows a few basic facts about the condition, she will not assume the role of the physician by giving medical advice, but she will be able to give understanding and reassurance that will support the medical therapy instead of undermining it.

A third area in which knowledge of facts may be important is in the follow-up period. If a student returns to college with an arrested case of tuberculosis, or to the elementary or secondary school with a heart defect, or a hearing or visual defect that has resulted from illness or accident, the health counselor can give understanding and support during the days of immediate adjustment and in the months ahead. Such support, based on scientific knowledge, may be extremely beneficial. The counselor who takes time to learn about the problems facing a student who must adjust to limitations can cooperate intelligently with all those who are trying to help in the total adjustment.

However, because in most cases the counselor confronted with health problems has a schedule that demands all of his time and energy, he cannot devote time to reading exhaustive books or articles about health conditions. It is with this in mind that the following two chapters have been written. They are limited in content, but they may point the direction that an interview should take and give some guidance as to when referral to a specialist is important. It is hoped that the counselor will use the references given at the end of each chapter to expand the scope of his knowledge as the need arises.

Bibliography

The following books and periodical references are recommended as good background material in the health area without specific reference to any one field of health.

Gordon, H. Phoebe, Katherine Densford, and E. G. Williamson, *Counseling in Schools of Nursing,* New York: McGraw-Hill, 1947.

Harrison, T. R., *Principles of Internal Medicine,* Philadelphia: The Blakiston Co., 1950, chapter 1.

Hiltner, Seward, *Pastoral Counseling,* New York-Nashville: Abingdon-Cokesbury Press, 1949. Attention is called to chapter 5, "Pastoral Counseling and Other Counseling," which suggests the need for the team-work approach in pastoral work.

Kirkpatrick, T. Bruce, "The Physical Education Teacher as Health Counselor," *The Journal-Lancet,* **60,** 451 (1940).

Nyswander, Dorothy B., *Solving School Health Problems,* the Astoria Demonstration Study, sponsored by the Department of Health and the Board of Education of New York City. Commonwealth Fund, 1942.

National Conference for Cooperation in Health Education, *Suggested School Health Policies,* New York: Health Education Council, 1946.

Smiley, Dean F., and Fred V. Hein, *Health Appraisal of School Children; Standards for Determining the Health Status of School Children—Through the Cooperation of Parents, Teachers, Physicians, Dentists, Nurses and Others:* A Report of the Joint Committee on Health Problems in Education of the National Education Association and the American Medical Association, 1948.

Tietz, Esther, and Martin Grotjahn, "Psychiatric Teamwork—An Integrated Therapy," *Journal of the American Medical Association,* **145,** 1057 (1951).

Wilson, Charles, "Health Counseling in Schools," *Public Health Nursing,* **37,** 436 (1945).

Wise, Carroll A., *Pastoral Counseling, Its Theory and Practice,* New York: Harper and Bros., 1951. An excellent discussion of counseling as it concerns pastors, with a recognition of the presence of health problems that may occur as part of the total need of the person seeking counsel.

Chapter IX

WHERE PHYSICAL SYMPTOMS PREDOMINATE

"My doctor prescribed pills containing iron, and told me to get plenty of sleep," Joan said to her teacher. Joan, a high school sophomore, had been feeling tired even when she started to school in the morning, and sometimes she had felt dizzy and things had gone black for a few seconds. She had not been interested in her lessons, and she had seemed irritable. She had always been a happy, enthusiastic student prior to the last few months.

Because of these changes in Joan, especially the fatigue and dizziness, her mother took her to their family physician. After reviewing Joan's past health and her present difficulties, the physician made a careful examination which included a chest X-ray and laboratory tests. The blood count showed that Joan had 3,600,000 red blood corpuscles and 9.75 grams of hemoglobin per 100 cubic centimeters of blood (equivalent to 65%). As a result of his findings, the physician made a diagnosis of secondary anemia.[1] He pursued his study further to determine why Joan was anemic so that he could correct the condition basically responsible for her symptoms. In the meantime, he prescribed medication indicated to meet existing body needs. He performed the information-giving

[1] The reader who is not familiar with medical terminology is referred to the Glossary.

function of the counselor when he said to Joan, "Take two pills after each meal," because he knew the need for medication and how large a dose was necessary to produce desired results. However he did not stop with this prescription for medicine. He engaged in health counseling by talking with Joan about her habits of sleep and diet. As a physician alert to Joan's emotions which would provide the necessary motivation, he did not say, "*Take* nine hours of sleep, and a diet with sufficient vitamins and minerals!" Instead, he took time to listen to Joan who brought up the question of sleep and diet, and together they talked about ways in which she could increase her hours of sleep, and improve her diet by increasing some of the important elements.

Joan's teacher had established a good relationship with her and as a result, Joan was anxious to explain why her grades had fallen down. The teacher became a part of the team. In the weeks that followed, she was able to give Joan understanding when she became tired and assurance that her work was satisfactory, so that Joan was able to go through the period of regaining her health without too much added tension or anxiety.

Joan was very fortunate because her doctor and teacher recognized the fact that every physical illness or abnormality has an emotional component. As Strecker has so strongly stated: "It is now clearly comprehended that an illness, any illness, even though it may appear to be restricted to the physical in its clinical expression, nevertheless, always contains a mental component which must be appreciated." [2] In Joan's illness physical symptoms predominated, but inescapably there followed emotional tensions. She had always been physically healthy. Did this illness mean that she would have to give up some of her dates or extracurricular activities? Could she still be on the basketball team? Why did she always feel so tired? Would she always have to force herself to do things? How

[2] Edward A. Strecker, *Fundamentals of Psychiatry,* 3rd Edition, Philadelphia: J. P. Lippincott Co., 1945, p. ix.

could she get her homework done when she had to get so much sleep? What if she failed in her exams? These and other questions forced themselves into her consciousness, but she learned to understand her illness and the reasons for her worries.

There are many such cases where the illness or defect is predominantly physical, but the emotional quality varies with each individual. One child who learns that he will have to adjust to a heart damaged by rheumatic fever will be resentful and bitter. Another will recognize the reality of the situation and try to find outlets for physical and emotional activity and creativity consistent with his limitations. The challenge to the health counselor is to help the child with the first reaction grow to the place where he will have the second reaction. In order to do this, the counselor must be familiar with a few basic facts so that he can be an intelligent listener when his client starts to talk about his particular problem, and so that any statements he may make will not be at variance with those of the physician or nurse. The conditions of physical illness or defect described on the following pages represent, in the experience of the authors, problems frequently present in health-counseling situations.[3] Those selected deal with: (1) problems of nutrition; (2) the skin, especially acne; (3) problems of hearing loss; (4) defects of vision; (5) cardiac conditions, especially rheumatic heart disease; (6) pulmonary conditions, especially tuberculosis; and (7) illnesses involving loss of consciousness and muscle coordination, especially epilepsy. In each of these areas, only those facts will be given which may aid the health counselor in his constant task of health education, in his role of screener for early referral to the physician, in his attempt to give intelligent support on the emotional level to the person receiving medical care, and in his share toward helping the client to adjust to his illness or defect in the rehabilitation period.

[3] The bibliography at the close of this chapter lists sources of information on other conditions.

Nutrition Problems

Good nutrition is not merely a matter of calories. If a student gets plenty of food and is not underweight, the teacher may not think of malnutrition when she sees that student in her classroom every day, even though he doesn't seem to have as much energy as the other boys.

Nutrition problems can arise whenever the food consumed or absorbed does not meet the body's needs. The following food needs of the body are suggested: (1) Leafy green or yellow vegetables—especially rich in vitamin A; (2) citrus fruit, tomato, or raw cabbage—rich in vitamin C; (3) potatoes, other vegetables, and fruits; (4) milk, cheese, ice-cream—rich in calcium and protein; (5) meat, poultry, fish, eggs, dried peas, beans—rich in protein; (6) bread, flour, and cereals—whole-grain or enriched—rich in vitamin B; and (7) butter or fortified margarines—rich in vitamins A and D. These foods should form the basis of the diet every day. The additional food needed by an individual will vary with his activities. The foods noted meet body needs by providing calories, vitamins, minerals, water, and the bulk essential to healthy intestinal action.

When deviations from normal arise in the field of nutrition, they can be expected to become evident through physical signs which result from a lack, or insufficient amount, of one or more of the basic food groups, and through emotional signs, such as irritability, and failure to cooperate or make social adjustments, which are the emotional components of physical illness. However, disturbances in the nutrition field may be subclinical, and only careful medical examination and laboratory tests will detect them. The health counselor cannot be expected to screen for a condition which as yet shows no outward symptoms. She can be aware of the possibility of such disturbance in the presence of unexplained physical or mental fatigue, and suggest that the student should see his physician. Where signs of disturbed nutrition do occur clinically, there are physical evidences. Let us look at some of the results of malnutrition.[4]

1. **Weight disturbances.** These disturbances are directly related to caloric intake in the absence of any disease which would prevent normal absorption of food through the intestinal wall. When, in the course of the day's activities, fewer calories are burned up to provide energy than are ingested, there will be a positive caloric balance, which is stored in the body and which results in overweight. In the words of L. H. Newburgh: "The simple principle (remains) that obesity is invariably the result of a disproportion between the inflow and the outflow of energy. The former must always be greater than the latter, either because the intake has increased, or the outgo has diminished." [5] In the same way, a negative caloric balance results in underweight.

The emotional component of weight, however, looms large in the picture. In the description of a case of an obese fifteen-year-old girl, the following statement is made: "There are two things of importance in this story. The patient arrived spontaneously at the decision to reduce and she had a very adequate reason which represented an approach to the problem of maturing. How successful she will be will not depend upon how well she remains on her diet, but rather on how well she will be able to develop satisfying human relationships." [6]

In this case, expert medical as well as psychological help may be necessary, but the health counselor who is not a clinical psychologist or psychiatrist may give support and help in the development of satisfying human relationships.

2. **Mineral and vitamin inadequacies.** The medical diagnosis of mineral and vitamin deficiencies is often difficult, because the clinical signs of such lacks in the diet appear only

[4] Malnutrition is defined as "imperfect nutrition" in Blakiston's *New Gould Medical Dictionary*, 1949.

[5] Norman Jolliffe, F. F. Tisdall, and Paul R. Cannon: *Clinical Nutrition*, New York: Paul B. Hoeber, 1950, p. 720.

[6] Flanders Dunbar, *Synopsis of Psychosomatic Diagnosis and Treatment*, St. Louis: C. V. Mosby Co., 1948, p. 260.

TABLE I

Minerals and Vitamins Important to the Growth and Function of the Human Body

Name	*Best Sources*	*Normal Uses*	*Results of Deficiency*
Calcium and phosphorus (usually in combination)	Milk; cheese	Formation and upkeep of bones and teeth	Poor bones and teeth
Iron	Eggs, meats, liver; green leaf vegetables	Essential in manufacture of hemoglobin	Anemia of iron deficiency type
Iodine	Sea food of all kinds	Essential in secretion of thyroid gland	Abnormal thyroid function; enlargement of gland
Sodium and chloride	Table salt	In blood; in gastric juice; in control of water balance	Loss of control of water passage into and out of tissues
Copper	Liver; nuts; dried legumes	Essential to use of iron in forming hemoglobin	Faulty formation of hemoglobin leading to anemia
Vitamin A	Butter; eggs; fish-liver oils; green leaf and yellow vegetables; peaches	Promotes growth; prevents infections of respiratory tract; vision in dim light; maintains healthy skin and mucous membranes	Poor bone structure and growth; frequent colds; nightblindness; infections of skin and mucous membranes
Vitamin B complex (thiamin, riboflavin, niacin, and other B factors)	Whole grains; lean meats; milk; egg yolks; oysters; green leaf vegetables; beans; peas	Vigor; good appetite and digestion; healthy nerves; growth	Neuritis; beri-beri; pellagra*
Vitamin C	Citrus fruits; tomatoes; green leaf vegetables	For good teeth and gums; upkeep of tissues	Scurvy*
Vitamin D	Ultraviolet rays of sun; fish liver oils; irradiated milk	Formation of bones and teeth; necessary for calcium utilization	Rickets*
Vitamin E	Wheat germ; green leaf vegetables; vegetable oils	Reproduction process; nerve and muscle functioning	Experimental in animals; no proved deficiency in man
Vitamin K	Green leaf vegetables; yellow vegetables; eggs	Necessary for clotting of blood	Delayed blood clotting, resulting in bleeding

* See Glossary.

after a period of poor nutrition where there has been a cumulative effect. Also, single vitamin deficiencies are rare. A well-rounded diet contains sufficient quantities of vitamins to meet the body's daily requirements. Deficiencies may result, especially in teen-age girls, from extreme and unbalanced diets. Vitamins may also be lacking because of improper preservation or preparation of green vegetables and other foods. The condensed list of table 1 of some of the minerals and vitamins that are vital to body growth and function may call the health counselor's attention to possible physical disturbances that may contribute to emotional maladjustments. It may also serve him in his information-giving function when he has no professional nutritionist at hand and problems of nutrition arise in the course of counseling.

A more complete study of the given ingredients and of others, such as vitamin B 12 and folic acid, may be found in books referred to in the bibliography at the end of this chapter.

The Skin: Acne[7]

While any blemish or lesion on a visible part of the skin produces an emotional component, the condition most frequently confronting the health counselor who works with adolescents is acne. Other skin conditions may be contagious, more disfiguring (the adolescent who is the sufferer may not agree), or even more resistant to treatment (again challenged by the client), but because acne occurs so frequently during the adolescent period that it is considered by some almost physiological, it has become a serious deterrent to happiness for many teen-agers.

Certain facts are generally known to teachers and others engaged in health counseling with this age group: That it occurs during puberty or the adolescent period of the vast majority of individuals; that it involves the hair follicles and oil glands

[7] The term, as used here, refers to the skin condition known medically as "acne vulgaris."

of the skin on the face, shoulders, chest, and back; that it may be very mild or so severe that it will produce permanent scarring; that no one specific cause has been found, although it is usually associated with adolescent glandular changes that result in increased activity of the oil glands of the skin; that it is linked, in some cases, with certain foods, such as chocolate; that no specific cure has been found; and that eventually it is self-limiting, disappearing in most cases during the late teens or early twenties.

Medical texts have little information to add that would be helpful to the health counselor. Recognition of acne is not difficult since it is based on: (1) age, (2) localization, (3) presence of comedones, and (4) history of the disease. For determination of the possible cause and for treatment, early referral to a physician is imperative, because untreated acne may last long and is more prone to leave permanent scarring. Treatment by the physician, preferably a skin specialist, centers around hygiene, including concern as to cosmetics used, local treatment for removal of blackheads, the application of a lotion suited to the individual case, X-ray in some severe cases, and dietary management that is aimed at avoiding foods with high oil or fat content. Other therapy may be necessary when the case is associated with anemia, vitamin lacks, weight disturbance, glandular disturbance, or constipation. Such medical treatment may eventually bring desired results. However, the adjustment by the student to the presence of this type of disfigurement at an age when both boys and girls want to be attractive to the opposite sex is a problem that can well challenge the patience and understanding of parents and teachers as well as physicians. In addition to giving the support the student needs, the health counselor can also help him to realize the inadequacy, and often the danger, of following the advice of well-meaning friends or magazine, radio, and television advertisements. A wonder drug or miracle cure may be found for acne through further medical research, but until such discovery is made and tested, the student may be led to recognize what is happening to him, where he can get the best scientific help, and how he can live with his acne until nature and the doctor can effect a cure.

Hearing Defects

The question as to whether hearing or sight is more important to the normal total adjustment of the individual is one that cannot be readily answered. Perhaps to most people loss of sight is the greatest threat they can imagine, but there are those who, if given a choice, would dread a loss of hearing more. They feel that, with physical vision gone, they would still have the whole world of music and the spoken word without which life would be barren. Whatever the answer for the individual, there can be unanimous agreement on the fact that hearing is a vital part of living and that partial or complete loss of hearing is a physical defect in which the emotional component approaches its height. Any defect that involves a limitation in the means of contacting one's environment becomes a threat which calls forth disturbing emotions. The hard-of-hearing child or adult tends to become irritable, shy, sullen, stubborn, or suspicious. He may receive excellent medical care by a physician who is interested in him as a whole individual and recognizes the emotional needs, but he does not see the physician frequently enough. He will be aided or hindered in his adjustment to his defect by the attitudes and actions of those whom he meets in his daily experiences. The person who has a counseling relationship with him can be especially helpful.

Before the hearing loss occurred, such a defect was not within the scope of the individual's comprehension. After it occurred, especially if the onset was rapid, he could not picture himself as being so handicapped. If he is to develop a mature adjustment, he must not only accept necessary medical treatment and learn to use a hearing aid if that is indicated; he must also learn to accept himself with his defect. He must come to the realization that the picture of himself as a person without perfect hearing is not intolerable. Only when he reaches this point can he live constructively. He may be able to arrive at this emotional adjustment by himself, or he may desperately need the support of a teacher, pastor, social worker, or professional counselor.

There are some medical facts regarding hearing loss that may help the counselor who is confronted with a problem involving this defect.

(1) **Types of hearing loss.** "There are two types of deafness. These are conduction deafness, in which the difficulty is in the middle ear, and nerve deafness, in which the difficulty is in the internal ear, cochlear nerve, or auditory center. . . . Individuals affected with conduction deafness can hear well through the bones of the skull, due to the fact that sound waves may be carried through bone.[8] . . . In nerve deafness there is no ability to hear in the advanced stages." [9]

(2) **How to detect hearing loss in the child: by observation; by tests.** A child who has had a hearing loss for a long period of time, perhaps since birth or early childhood when it followed an acute ear infection, has no basis of comparison for knowing that he does not hear well. The alert teacher, however, may become aware of the child's difficulty through daily observations. The child may turn his head slightly when spoken to. His voice may sound flat and unnatural. He may be inattentive when class directions are given out or when he is not looking at the speaker. He may watch the teacher closely in order to understand him better through interpreting his movements or through conscious or unconscious lip reading. He may constantly ask for repetition of questions. He may try to copy assignments for home work from his neighbor. He may fail to answer easy questions.

The teacher, nurse, or health educator may also detect hearing loss by means of tests. Those tests which are widely

[8] The appliances for deaf individuals are so arranged as to make use of this fact.

[9] Esther M. Greisheimer, *Physiology and Anatomy,* 5th Edition, Philadelphia: J. B. Lippincott Co., 1945, p. 371.

accepted at present are the whisper test for rough screening purposes, the group audiometer test for more scientific screening, and the individual pitch tone audiometer test for determination of degree and range of hearing loss. More detailed descriptions of these tests are available from agencies concerned with the prevention of hearing loss.[10]

The administration of these tests is not part of the counseling procedure, but an understanding of the reports made on the basis of the tests may be very useful.

(*a*) *The whisper test.* The results of this test are expressed as a fraction, the number of feet of distance between tester and child being the numerator, and 20 feet—the distance at which he should be able to hear the whispered voice—being the denominator. Thus, right 10/20, left 20/20 would indicate that the child could hear the whisper with his right ear only when he was 10 feet from the tester instead of the normal distance of 20 feet. Such a child should be referred for a more valid test.

(*b*) *The group audiometer test.* A hearing loss becomes apparent through this test because the child who listens through ear phones to the numbers announced from the recording in a voice that gradually decreases in intensity fails to hear some of the numbers. Evidence of any hearing loss by this method should lead to referral of the child for an individual pitch tone audiometer test.

(*c*) *Pitch tone audiometer test.* This test consists of checking each ear through ear phones by pitch tones from low to high frequency with increasing intensity of sound. The point of intensity at which each sound is heard is recorded on a graph. The report is given in terms of decibels of hearing loss. Decibel is the unit of loudness, the word being compounded from the Latin decimus and the name of Alexander Graham Bell, inventor of the telephone. Children showing a hearing loss of 12 decibels or more in either ear are examined

[10] The American Hearing Society, 1537 Thirty-fifth Street, N. W., Washington, D. C.

by an otologist. This examination will discover such conditions as an excessive collection of wax in the ear, middle ear disease, nose and throat disease with thickening of the Eustachian tube, or the presence of nerve deafness. If the pitch tone test shows a loss of 20 decibels or more in the better ear, the child may be recommended by the otologist for a hearing aid, mouth-reading instruction, or for instruction in a special school.

(3) **Ways of treating hearing loss.** When the cause has been determined by otological examination and audiometer testing, any local condition is treated medically or surgically to obtain the best possible results. In cases of the conductive type of deafness, a hearing aid may be recommended. Other modern methods for improving hearing through surgery are constantly being developed.

Defects of Vision

It might be assumed that what has been said regarding hearing loss could be paralleled and applied to the loss of vision. There is, however, a difference in the areas where health counseling is most applicable. In the field of visual defects which cause partial loss or distortion of vision, there is less emotional tension because the wearing of glasses to correct eyesight is so common an occurrence. The wearing of glasses is accepted by individuals, even teen-agers, since modern design and varied colors have brought glamor to the staid spectacles of grandmother's day. Science has produced in recent years the contact lens, and now for use in selected cases the corneal lens, which defies detection. Glasses are also accepted by society. A college graduate who wears glasses is not afraid that this will prevent him from obtaining a desired job except in the case of a few very exacting occupations. If, however, he wears a hearing aid, this may detract greatly from his employability. There are still many boards of education which raise no objection to poor vision that is correctible by proper lenses, but which will not license a young teacher who has more than a 10 per cent hearing loss even though his hearing can be made adequate by the use of a hearing aid.

The vital importance of vision, however, in the individual's total adjustment to his world makes advisable a consideration of a few basic facts about visual defects.

(1) **Causes of defective vision.** A person may have difficulty in seeing with one or both eyes because of deviation from normal in the shape of the eyeball, the surface of the lens or cornea, the functioning of eye muscles, or because of disease of the eye.

If the eyeball is too long or too short, the image of a perceived object is brought to focus in front of or behind the retina, with a resultant blurring of the image at the place where the light rays impinge on the retina. When the eyeball is too long, the defect is called myopia or nearsightedness which can be corrected by the use of a concave lens of suitable strength. When the eyeball is too short, the condition is called hyperopia or farsightedness and a convex lens must be used for correction. A defect in the surface of the eye lens or cornea which produces an irregularity of light refraction, again resulting in a blurred image, is called astigmatism. This can be corrected by cylindrical lenses set at the proper angle to overcome the differences in curvature of the surfaces involved. If one of the muscles controlling the movements of the eye is weak, there will be muscle imbalance and strabismus, or cross-eye, will result.

(2) **Signs of defective vision.** There are signs which may be observed by a teacher or parent; the child or adult with vision defect may complain and screening tests may be made to detect abnormalities.

Holding books too close or beyond the usual distance, mistaking letters or figures, tilting the head, frowning while reading, misreading work on the blackboard, rubbing the eyes, inability to move the eyes together, repeated failure to catch a ball thrown from a distance in outdoor play—these are things a teacher can observe. Dizziness, headache, nausea, blurred vision, sensitiveness to light, a feeling of sand in the eyes—these are complaints made by the child. Crustiness of eyelids, redness of or discharge from the eyes, the presence of sties—these are evidences of chronic or acute eye infection. Reading from a Snellen chart at a distance of 20 feet in good light which comes from the side is a screening test that may be made by a classroom or health education teacher.

(3) **The health counselor's responsibility.** A counselor, being aware of possible deviations from normal vision, should be alert to notice signs of such difficulty. Unrecognized poor vision may be a contributing cause of emotional disturbances. The counselor should make early referral to a physician if this is indicated. He may help the teen-ager to recognize the importance of wearing glasses as prescribed by the eye specialist. In cases where sight is threatened or where there is partial or complete blindness, he can create the kind of counseling relationship that will enable the client to adjust to the reality of this very serious handicap.

Rheumatic Fever

The story of medical understanding of disease during the last two centuries is a fascinating one. It might be likened to the solving of a giant jig-saw puzzle. Pieces that look unrelated because of variations in color and design may prove to be parts of a cottage that is a clearly defined entity in the completed picture. Before the basic cause of a disease was known, physicians recognizing a group of symptoms that seemed to occur together classified them as a disease. Another group of symptoms would be labelled as a different disease. Through medical research, there has gradually evolved a recognition of the relatedness of some of these disease entities and the puzzle has begun to take shape. Such was the case with syphilis. This contagious disease has been known for centuries, but many of its manifestations were not recognized as part of the disease until the spirochete, which is the cause of syphilis, was discovered at the beginning of this century and its action on tissues learned through a study of pathology. Then some cases of heart disease, types of mental illness, or cases of motor paralysis affecting the legs, which might have appeared years following a latent period when there were no obvious symptoms, were found to be due to the same spirochete affecting various tissues of the body. At last, the jig-saw puzzle was completed. Our modern concept of syphilis emerged.

Our present concept of rheumatic fever has likewise been put together as the relatedness of several aspects of the disease has emerged from medical research. Rheumatic fever is an acute disease that usually starts with a sore throat and spreads to the joints, causing an acute inflammation there and producing a fever that may last for weeks. It may develop complications which, at one time, were not recognized as part of the whole rheumatic fever picture. One of these is chorea, known as St. Vitus' dance, and another is rheumatic heart disease. It is this last condition which accounts for more than 80 per cent of the heart disease found in young adults and which is responsible for most of the deaths resulting from rheumatic fever.

The importance of early discovery and treatment of the disease and of the prevention of recurrences is widely recognized. What facts about rheumatic fever can aid the health counselor?

(1) **Cause.** The exact cause of rheumatic fever is not known, but in a susceptible individual, an attack is frequently preceded by a streptococcal infection, such as a bad cold, tonsillitis, or scarlet fever. The susceptibility referred to seems to be connected with damp and overcrowded living quarters, a poor diet, or a possible hereditary factor. Although the disease is due to an infection, it is not passed from one child to another through contact. One case in a classroom does not result in an epidemic.

(2) **Early signs of rheumatic fever.** The first attack most frequently occurs between the ages of 5 and 12. The evidences

of actual illness are often vague. Failure to gain weight, poor appetite, fatigue, persistent low fever, repeated nosebleeds, and emotional disturbances, such as irritability and crying spells without good reason, may be symptoms. Painful or sore and inflamed joints are a more definite sign of the disease, and are responsible for the term "rheumatic" in its name. Emotional disturbances and uncontrollable twitching and jerking of the face, arms, and legs may indicate the development of chorea, the effect of rheumatic fever on the nervous system. Development of rheumatic heart disease as the streptococcus attacks the lining of the heart (endocardium) is discovered through careful heart study by the physician. The heart may be temporarily affected and may completely recover, or may receive permanent damage, especially of the leaflets of one or more of the four valves of the heart.

(3) **To what must the child or adolescent adjust?** There are at least three factors to which the child suffering from rheumatic fever must make an emotional adjustment. In some cases there will be a fourth.

(a) As soon as a diagnosis is made, and early diagnosis is of utmost importance if a favorable prognosis is expected, the child must have complete bed rest. This means that at the age when most children enjoy physical activity, and have opportunities to satisfy their curiosity about the world they live in, the rheumatic fever child must lie in bed for weeks and months, getting his satisfaction from pictures, books, or toys which require little physical effort for their enjoyment. This condition is further aggravated by the fact that the majority of cases occur in overcrowded, low-income groups where money for books, toys, record-players, and radios is nonexistent and where the mother has little leisure time to read to or play with her child.

(b) The convalescent period is prolonged so that when the child is allowed out of bed, he must learn to go slowly in his journey back to the normal, and children do not, of their own accord, go slowly.

(c) Because recurrences are a constant threat,[11] he must have regular check-ups by a physician. He must learn to avoid precipitating causes of recurrence, such as undue exposure to rain and cold, contact with other children who have nose and throat infections, and fatigue from insufficient rest. All of these things make the child feel different from the rest of his group.

(d) When the heart valves are permanently damaged by the streptococcus that is active in rheumatic fever, the involvement may be so mild that the child need have no restrictions, or so severe that he must remain in bed or chair. The degree of necessary emotional adjustment in such cases will cover a wide scale. The American Heart Association has adopted standards as an indication for the amount of activity a child with rheumatic heart disease can engage in without further injury to the heart. These standards or classes, which are given in the following list, are used by physicians in advising school personnel.

(1) Patients with heart disease whose physical activity need not be restricted.

(2) Patients with heart disease whose ordinary physical activity need not be restricted, but who should be advised against unusually severe or competitive sports.

(3) Patients with heart disease whose ordinary physical activities should be moderately restricted and whose more strenuous habitual efforts should be discontinued.

(4) Patients with heart disease whose ordinary physical activity should be markedly restricted.

(5) Patients with heart disease who should be at complete rest, confined to bed or chair. (Of patients who have had rheumatic heart disease, only about 15 per cent have to limit drastically their activity.)

[11] Although the sulfa drugs have not proved useful in treatment of rheumatic fever, in recent years, there were fewer recurrences when small doses were given over long periods of time under the close supervision of a physician. Their use cannot be indiscriminate, but there is a promise of greater control of recurrences through their action.

The greatest need for wise counseling arises in the child or teen-ager during this rehabilitation period. Tom, a high school sophomore, had rheumatic fever when he was eight but it did not damage his heart, and he is now well on the way to becoming the star tackle for his football team. Then he has a recurrence of rheumatic fever. He is in bed for four months. This time, the heart valves are damaged and he develops a leakage of the valve between the right auricle and ventricle. He is classified in group 3, and he returns to school in his junior year with the realization that he will have to play football vicariously, from the sidelines. The teacher who can help Tom grow beyond his initial resentment and bitterness to the place where he can accept his defect and find satisfying outlets consistent with it will be filling one of the most important roles in health counseling.

The other side of the picture must also be strongly stressed. When the physician places a child in class 1, the teacher can be of great assistance in encouraging the child to adjust to his health status. The discipline of months of bed rest, together with the reactions of an overly cautious and fear-ridden mother, may result in unnecessary physical and emotional invalidism. It may be almost as difficult to help the child grow from a position where he is dependent, fearful, and controlled by a feeling of physical inferiority, to a position where he can become independent, confident, and sure of his place in the groups to which he belongs.

Tuberculosis

"Where physical symptoms predominate!" Where indeed do they predominate more than in tuberculosis? It is a contagious disease caused by bacilli that can invade almost any part of the body, although their first line of attack is usually the respiratory system. The germs destroy normal lung tissue and produce serious illness, which may result in death. The cause, the symptoms, and the effects of the disease, all seem to be in the realm of physical medicine. The physician and nurse are the specialists trained to deal with such a condition. Are there facts indicating the need for a health-counseling team?

(1) **Diagnosis of pulmonary tuberculosis.** Skin tests for tuberculosis can be made to show that at some time the tuberculosis germ has entered the body causing a primary infection in the lymph glands around the bronchial tubes. These tests are the Patch test, in which a small amount of tuberculin is applied to the skin on a patch of gauze, and the Mantoux test, in which a minute dose of tuberculin is injected into the skin. They are called tuberculin tests.

A chest X-ray will reveal changes in the lung tissue. This is used on all persons who show a positive tuberculin test and, in many schools, it is employed instead of a tuberculin test. In some colleges, both tuberculin tests and chest X-rays are made. The tuberculin test result will help determine the origin of lung tissue change observed in the X-ray, but the X-ray may also reveal nontuberculous pathology of heart, lung, or bony structure. In persons showing a suspicious lung lesion, an examination of sputum may demonstrate the presence of tuberculosis bacilli in many cases. If this test is negative, the germs may be found in material washed from the stomach.

(2) **Prevention of tuberculosis.** Because the specific cause of the disease is known, as well as its means of transmission by direct contact with droplets discharged during coughing, or with contaminated eating utensils and other articles used by a patient, much of the control program is in the field of prevention. The finding of every active case and the provision for treatment until the disease becomes inactive or arrested, offers our best means of prevention at the present time. This has been done with increasing success over the last half century through skin testing, mass civilian X-rays, and, recently, through the practice of obtaining chest X-rays of every patient admitted to a hospital. The unrecognized case of active tuberculosis constitutes the chief menace to nurses, doctors, and

other hospital personnel. BCG vaccine is being used in controlled groups with the hope that it will increase the body's defenses against infection, but its use must still be considered experimental, although in many European countries, it is being used on a much wider scale.

Rigorous tuberculin testing of cattle and pasteurization of milk supplies has almost eliminated infection with the bovine type of tuberculosis, which formerly caused many cases among infants and small children.

(3) **Early signs of tuberculosis.** These have become generally known through extensive public health education. The fact that most cases of tuberculosis do not show clinical symptoms until the disease has passed the minimal stage must be stressed. Routine tuberculin testing and X-rays will reveal the minimal lesion which represents the early stage when treatment is most successful. At the same time, there is need for awareness of physical signs of the disease, since the general population does not as yet participate in a complete control program, and many cases advance to a more serious stage without detection by the methods mentioned. Such signs might be listed as unexplained weight loss, the persistence of a chronic cough after a chest cold, fatigue, and general loss of interest in work and play. These signs of illness are indefinite, but they indicate a need for a complete diagnostic study if they persist or progress.

(4) **Emotional aspects of tuberculosis.** The foundation stone of the treatment of active tuberculosis is rest: rest in bed for the whole individual, and frequently rest for the involved lung by injection of air into the chest cavity which is called pneumothorax. This causes temporary collapse of the lung with resulting rest for the tissues and greater opportunity of healing. Modern advances in the treatment of tuberculosis, including more extensive surgery and the use of streptomycin, do not eliminate the need for rest.

This prolonged rest period brings with it emotional tensions. Missing a year at school, cessation of normal social relationships for the high school or college student, socio-economic problems for the adult, and fear resulting from the ideas of tuberculosis that still exist in the average citizen's mind are all factors that contribute to these tensions. Tuberculosis is no longer a disease of youth alone. An increasingly large number of those of middle and advanced age groups have had reactivation of old, healed lesions, or a reinfection superimposed on a primary type of the disease. The social worker, clergyman, professional counselor, and teacher should develop the modern concept of tuberculosis if they are to help those with arrested tuberculosis adjust to such tensions. Tuberculosis *can* be found in its early stages: we have the diagnostic tools. It can be arrested: we have advanced methods of treatment. The individual who has had the disease can return to a normal, useful life, even to the extent of marrying and having a family: we have rehabilitation teams. Agencies will help with social and economic problems. Energy consumed in emotional conflict is lost to other bodily functions; it is lost to the body attempting to heal tuberculosis lesions. That is why the modern tuberculosis hospital has a team at work to meet the total needs of the patient, a team which includes the physician, nurse, psychologist, social worker, occupational therapist, and rehabilitation expert. They are all constantly assuming the role of health counselors in the hospital. When the student returns to school, or the adult to his job, the need for understanding and support is still there. Members of the family, pastor, or teacher may assume a health counselor's role.

Epilepsy

The term epilepsy is derived from a Greek word meaning seizure. Thus any seizure, or body convulsion, comes within the scope of epilepsy. Some cases of epilepsy originate in an organic cause, such as brain injury at birth or by an accident later in life, or a brain tumor. These are classified as *symptomatic* epilepsy because the seizure is a symptom of an underlying pathological condition. Other cases have not been shown to be associated with any organic lesion and are classified as *idiopathic* epilepsy. Whatever the classification, the person who has this disease needs help. He needs information that will supplant for him the many misconceptions that may have become rooted in his mind, such as, that epilepsy is a condition to be ashamed of and its presence in a family hidden from public knowledge, or that an epileptic person is feeble-minded. He needs to develop a sense of security and confidence. He is often rejected emotionally by family and friends. He finds himself questioned in school; his acceptance at many colleges is doubtful. He is unable to find employment, or he is employed with restrictions, such as avoidance of working near moving machinery, on high platforms or buildings, or of operating elevators, that limit his opportunity for advancement. These job restrictions are a necessary part of a safety program, but they result in a sense of frustration for the individual so restricted. The counselor who gives information and emotional help can do so more intelligently if he is familiar with some of the aspects of the disease.

(1) **Description of epilepsy.** Epilepsy is a disease characterized by seizures. A seizure is a temporary loss or impairment of consciousness which is usually accompanied by muscular movements which may range from a slight twitching of the eyelids to a violent shaking of the whole body. There are several types of epilepsy, the two most often referred to being grand mal and petit mal. In a grand mal seizure, the patient loses consciousness and falls, and twitches violently for a minute or two. He then relaxes and may get up, although he feels dull for a short period of time, or he may sleep for several hours. In a petit mal seizure, an attack lasts only a few seconds and is often overlooked. The patient rarely falls and there may be only a twitching of eyelids or eyebrows. This type may eventually disappear, or it may develop into grand mal epilepsy.

Epileptics are mentally normal people. Except for the occurrence of seizures, they are average human beings. They may have physical or mental illnesses as do nonepileptics, and where mental deficiency exists, it is coincidental with the epilepsy except in those cases where a brain disease or tumor may interfere with normal mental functioning.

(2) **Cause of epilepsy.** The ultimate factor in epilepsy, as in many other diseases, is a predisposition or a susceptibility to it. How large a part inheritance plays in this susceptibility is a debatable point. According to some studies made in recent years, the chance that a child of average parents will be epileptic is one in two hundred, while the chance that a child of an epileptic parent will be epileptic is one in forty.[12] A recording of the electrical waves given off by the brain, with the help of an instrument called the electro-encephalograph, may be helpful in recognizing a predisposition to epilepsy, for the brain wave patterns of most persons subject to seizures are different from those of most healthy persons. However, while one person in ten has some irregularity of the brain wave pattern, only one person in every two hundred has seizures. There must be more than a predisposition to epilepsy to produce the clinical evidence of seizures.

When a predisposition exists, many factors may produce an actual seizure. Some of these appear to be brain injury or disease, an illness or disorder elsewhere in the body, and emotional maladjustments. The maladjustments do not have to be in the form of external emotional crises. Some recent studies have suggested that petit mal attacks may occur as a psychosomatic symptom of a disturbance caused by a life situation. In a petit mal patient who was studied intensively there was evidence that an attack occurred as a specific response within the central nervous system which abolished consciousness when her pattern of integration was threatened

[12] Herbert Yahraes, *Epilepsy—the Ghost Is Out of the Closet,* Public Affairs Pamphlet Number 98, New York: Public Affairs Committee, Inc., 1945.

by a discrepancy between her consciously acceptable responses and her true unconscious reactions.[13]

(3) **First aid care during a grand mal seizure is important.** In a classroom, an epileptic child should be seated near the teacher's desk. If an attack occurs, the teacher should try to prevent the child from hitting his head as he falls and should then keep the child on the floor. A tongue depressor or pencil wrapped in a clean handkerchief should be placed between the teeth so that the tongue will not be bitten. After the seizure, the child should be allowed to rest where he will not be in a draft.

(4) **How the physician treats epilepsy.** If seizures are found to be due to a brain lesion, surgery may eliminate the cause. In general, good hygiene and correction of any existing physical defect is important.

Medical treatment offers the greatest control of the seizures at the present time. The drugs used are designed to lessen the number and severity of the seizures, or to stop them altogether. Each case must be studied individually to determine the right drug or combination of drugs that will most effectively control the seizures with the fewest harmful effects, such as nausea or skin eruptions. The drugs most frequently used are phenobarbital, dilantin, and tridione. They must be taken daily over long periods of time and must be given under careful medical supervision. Research workers are trying to find other drugs that will reduce the number and severity of seizures even more drastically than the ones in use, without causing harmful effects.

(5) **Emotional aspects.** Many emotional disturbances are an indirect result of seizures rather than a cause. The epileptic person develops feelings of insecurity, shyness, or often aggressiveness as a defense mechanism, not because it is part

[13] Wayne Barker, "Studies in Epilepsy: The Petit Mal Attack as a Response within the Central Nervous System to Distress in Organism-environment Integration," *Psychosomatic Medicine,* Vol. X, No. 2, March-April 1948.

of the disease, but because of the failure of his family, friends, and society to accept him as a person who is normal and healthy except for the handicap of his seizures. This handicap may become a very minor one under experienced medical care. He may attend regular school if his seizures can be kept under moderate control; he can engage in physical activities; he can hold a job; he can marry and have children. The extent to which he can do each of these things will depend on his particular case, and his doctor will guide him in these spheres.

The health counselor who accepts an epileptic person as a normal individual and who is aware of the great advance that has been made in the understanding and control of epileptic seizures will contribute greatly to the prevention of or adjustment to emotional disturbances that result from epilepsy.

Summary

The deviations from health described in this chapter have been offered as those typical of the problems arising in health counseling situations. Many more could have been discussed. Poliomyelitis, cancer, and veneral disease create serious emotional problems. Facts about them, however, are widely known through public health education, magazine articles, and pamphlets published by agencies created to deal specially with their prevention and treatment.

It is hoped that the information given will not only aid the health counselor as he deals with the specific illnesses mentioned, but also will suggest to him a way to approach other problems of similar nature. Familiarity with causes, recognition of early signs, awareness of possible outcomes with needs for rehabilitation or redirection of energies are all important tools in the hands of the person who counsels in health situations. Some knowledge of methods of treatment gives the health counselor assurance that he may encourage a feeling of hope and dispel despair in certain problems. An example of this is the present picture of meningitis, the mention of which twenty years ago brought great alarm. Today, there is no reason for panic if early diagnosis is made and treatment given with one of the sulfa drugs or an antibiotic. Similar information on other diseases may be obtained from many sources: pamphlets, such as those published by the Public Affairs Committee, books on personal and community health, health education departments of boards of health, or agencies dealing with specific health problems. In addition, there is always the physician who, if he realizes that you are a person qualified to counsel intelligently and wisely, will welcome you to the team that is interested in the physical and emotional well-being of the patient.

Bibliography

General

American Association of School Administrators, *Health in Schools, 20th Yearbook,* Washington, D. C.: American Association of School Administrators, 1942.

Cannon, W. B., "The Influence of the Emotional States on the Functions of the Alimentary Tract," *American Journal of the Medical Sciences,* 137, 483 (1909).

Committee on Educational Adaptations for Children with Special Problems, *Children with Special Health Problems,* New York: National Tuberculosis Association, 1948.

Davison, Wilburt C., *The Compleat Pediatrician,* Durham, N. C.: Duke University Press, 1946.

Dunbar, Flanders, *Synopsis of Psychosomatic Diagnosis and Treatment,* St. Louis: the C. V. Mosby Co., 1948. Written for physicians; a guidebook in newer methods of diagnosis and treatment, especially those methods that are applicable to the patients who present the physician with baffling problems.

Etheredge, Maude L., *Health Facts for College Students,* Philadelphia: W. B. Saunders Co., 1947.

Gallagher, J. Roswell, *You and Your Health,* Life Adjustment Booklet, Chicago: Science Research Associates, 1951.

Goldberger, I, and Grace Hallock, *Understanding Health,* New York: Ginn and Co., 1950.

Grout, Ruth E., *Health Teaching in Schools,* Philadelphia: W. B. Saunders Co., 1949. See chapter 10, "Coworkers in Health Education."

Harrison, T. R., *Principles of Internal Medicine,* Philadelphia: The Blakiston Co., 1950.

Jones, H. W., et al, *Blakiston's New Gould Medical Dictionary,* 1st Edition, Philadelphia: The Blakiston Co., 1949.

Leonard, Margaret, *Health Counseling for Girls,* New York: A. S. Barnes and Co., 1944.

Meredith, Florence, *Health and Fitness,* Boston: D. C. Heath and Co., 1946.

Morrison, W. R., and L. B. Chenoweth, *Normal and Elementary Physical Diagnosis,* Philadelphia: Lea and Febiger, 1947.

Mustard, Harry S., *An Introduction to Public Health,* 2nd Edition, New York: The Macmillan Co., 1948. Information on diseases and health problems that are the concern of the community, such as, tuberculosis, communicable diseases of childhood, cancer, and heart disease.

Neugarten, Bernice L., *Your Heredity,* Life Adjustment Booklet, Chicago: Science Research Associates.

Rogers, James Frederick, *What Every Teacher Should Know about the Physical Condition of Her Pupils,* Pamphlet No. 68 (revised 1945), Washington, D. C.: Federal Security Agency, U. S. Office of Education.

Third National Conference on Health in Colleges, *A Health Program for Colleges,* New York: National Tuberculosis Assoc., 1948.

Turner, C. E., *Personal and Community Hygiene,* 7th Edition, St. Louis: The C. V. Mosby Co., 1943.

Turner, C. E., *School Health and Health Education,* St. Louis: The C. V. Mosby Co., 1947.

Weiss, Edward, and O. Spurgeon English, *Psychosomatic Medicine,* Philadelphia: W. B. Saunders Co., 1943.

Wolf, S., and H. G. Wolff, "Life Situations; Emotions and Gastric Function; A Summary," *American Practitioner,* Vol. III, No. 1, Sept. 1948.

Allergies

U. S. Public Health Service, *Hay Fever and Asthma,* Leaflet, Washington, D. C.: U. S. Public Health Service.

Anatomy and Physiology

Best, Charles Herbert, and Norman Burke Taylor, *The Living Body; a Text in Human Physiology,* Revised Edition, New York: Henry Holt, 1944.

Greisheimer, Esther M., *Physiology and Anatomy,* 5th Edition, Philadelphia: J. B. Lippincott Co., 1945.

Cancer

Johnson, Dallas, *Facing the Facts about Cancer,* Public Affairs Pamphlet No. 38, New York: Public Affairs Committee, Inc., 2nd Edition, 1948.

Communicable Diseases

American Public Health Association, *The Control of Communicable Diseases in Man,* 7th Edition, New York: The American Public Health Association, 1950.

Chadwick, Henry Dexter, and Alton S. Pope, *The Modern Attack on Tuberculosis,* New York: Commonwealth Fund, 1946.

National Tuberculosis Association, *Tuberculosis, a Manual for Teachers,* New York: National Tuberculosis Association, 1947.

National Tuberculosis Association, *TB through the Teens,* New York: National Tuberculosis Association, 1946.

Diabetes

Anon., *Concerning Diabetes,* Leaflet, Boston: John Hancock Life Insurance Co., 1946.

Anon., *Diabetes Mellitus,* Leaflet, Washington, D. C.: U. S. Public Health Service.

Epilepsy

Barker, Wayne, "Studies in Epilepsy: The Petit Mal Attack as a Response within the Central Nervous System to Distress in Organism-environment Integration," *Psychosomatic Medicine,* Vol. X, No. 2, March-April 1948.

Lennox, William G., *Science and Seizures: New Light on Epilepsy and Migraine,* New York: Harper and Bros., 1941.

Yahraes, Herbert, *Epilepsy—the Ghost Is Out of the Closet,* Public Affairs Pamphlet No. 98, New York: Public Affairs Committee, Inc., 1945.

Handicapped

Dobbins, E. C., and Ruth Abernathy, *Physical Education Activities for Handicapped Children,* New York: University of the State of New York, 1937.

Hamilton, Kenneth W., *Counseling the Handicapped in the Rehabilitation Process,* New York: The Ronald Press Co., 1950.

Mackie, Romaine P., *Crippled Children in School,* Washington, D. C.: Federal Security Agency, 1948.

Pintner, R., J. Eisenson, and M. Stanton, *The Psychology of the Physically Handicapped,* New York: F. S. Crofts Co., 1945.

Taylor, Eugene J., *Help at Last for the Cerebral Palsy,* Public Affairs Pamphlet No. 158, New York: Public Affairs Committee, Inc., 1950.

Heart Conditions

Blakeslee, Howard, *Know Your Heart,* Public Affairs Pamphlet No. 137, 2nd Edition, New York: Public Affairs Committee, Inc., 1949.

Anon., *The Cardiac Child in School and Community,* New York: The New York Heart Association, March 1949.

U. S. Children's Bureau, *Facts about Rheumatic Fever,* Publication No. 297, Washington, D. C.: Federal Security Agency.

Haseltine, N. S., *The Human Heart,* Washington, D. C.: Superintendent of Documents, U. S. Government Printing Office, 1950.

Joint Report of Committee on School Health and Rheumatic Fever of the American Academy of Pediatrics, "Rheumatic Fever and the School Child," *New York Medicine,* March 5, 1949.

Yahraes, Herbert, *Rheumatic Fever; Childhood's Greatest Enemy.* Public Affairs Pamphlet No. 126, New York: Public Affairs Committee, Inc., 3rd Edition, 1949.

Human Development

Biester, Lillian L., William Griffiths, and N. O. Pearce, *Units in Personal Health and Human Relations,* Minneapolis: University of Minnesota Press, 1947.

Fedder, Ruth, *A Girl Grows Up,* 2nd Edition, New York: McGraw-Hill, 1948.

Fields, Morey K., J. A. Goldberg, and H. F. Kilander, *Youth Grows into Adulthood,* New York: Chartwell House, 1950.

Kirkendall, Lester A., *Understanding Sex,* Chicago: Science Research Association, 1948.

Lloyd-Jones, Esther, and Ruth Fedder, *Coming of Age,* New York: McGraw-Hill, 1941.

McKown, Harry C., *A Boy Grows Up,* New York: McGraw-Hill, 1949.

Narcotics and Stimulants

Fields, Morey K., *Symposium on Alcohol Education,* New York: New York University School of Education, 1948.

Merrill, Frederick T., *Marihuana,* The New Dangerous Drug, Washington, D. C.: Opium Research Committee, Foreign Policy Association, 1941.

Steinhaus, Arthur H., and Florence M. Grunderman, *Tobacco and Health,* 4th Edition, New York: Association Press, 1948.

Yahraes, Herbert, *Alcoholism Is a Sickness,* Public Affairs Pamphlet No. 118, New York: Public Affairs Committee, Inc., 1950.

Nutrition

Cooper, Lenna Frances, Edith Michael, and Helen Swift Mitchell, *Nutrition in Health and Disease,* 10th Edition, Philadelphia: J. B. Lippincott Co., 1947.

Joliffe, Norman, E. F. Tisdall, and Paul R. Cannon, *Clinical Nutrition,* New York: Paul B. Hoeber, Inc., 1950.

Skin Diseases

Tobias, Norman, *Essentials of Dermatology,* Philadelphia: J. B. Lippincott Co., 1945.

Vision

Foote, F. M., "Milestones in Sight Conservation," *The Yale Journal of Biology and Medicine,* Vol. 19, No. 4, March 1947.

Hathaway, Winifred, *Education and Health of the Partially Seeing Child,* New York: Columbia University Press, Revised 1948.

Yahraes, Herbert, *What Do You Know About Blindness?* Public Affairs Pamphlet No. 124, New York: Public Affairs Committee, Inc., 1947.

Chapter X

WHERE EMOTIONAL SYMPTOMS PREDOMINATE

In the physical, or somatic[1] area of medicine, warnings that a doctor is needed are usually not too difficult to recognize. A mother notices that her baby's skin feels warm. She takes his temperature and finds that it is 100.5°F by rectal thermometer, which is equivalent to 99.5° F, as registered by the adult mouth thermometer. The baby does not want his milk and is fretful. The average mother does not call her doctor immediately at such a time unless other symptoms are present. She rechecks his temperature in an hour and watches him more carefully. If she finds that his temperature is rising, that he seems to be breathing more rapidly, that he vomits, or any one of a number of such things, she does not waste time watching her baby. She calls a doctor. Likewise, if, especially during an epidemic of measles, a teacher notices a fourth-grade child who is inattentive, has watery eyes and running nose, or is coughing, she does not keep him in class to watch him. She refers the child for medical attention. Physical symptoms can usually be seen, heard, observed through actions, or in some way measured, and warnings heeded.

In the area of emotional problems, the situation is not so simple. There are at least two reasons for this. First, be-

[1] The reader who is not familiar with medical terminology is referred to the Glossary.

cause we all have signs of emotional disturbances without considering ourselves abnormal, we are not likely to be sensitive to early signs of emotional and mental illness. We have all had a display of temper, or a period of depression when nothing seemed worth doing, or a period of unusual excitement when we could laugh, sing, or even cry on some small pretense. These are all considered normal aspects of human living. Second, because the history of medicine in the mental field is comparatively short, we have not as yet developed sufficient tools or techniques for the satisfactory measurement of disturbances in this area. We cannot place a thermometer in a high school student's mouth and learn whether or not his aggressive tendencies have gone above normal. In view of these facts, it is difficult for a health counselor to screen clients for referral to a specialist.

One must admit the risk involved in giving information concerning mental illness in a text such as this which is limited in size and which is for counselors who are not specialists in the field of medicine. If the classroom teacher, for example, is given a little knowledge about mental illness, will she not tend to categorize her student, to decide that he must be a schizophrenic because he fits the text-book picture so perfectly? The risk is there, but how much greater is the risk of missing the opportunity of securing help for the student while there is time. The well-trained health counselor will be aware of his limitations, but he will also be alert to repeated abnormalities in adjustment that he has an opportunity to observe. This will occur, in many cases, long before there has been any thought of referral in the minds of those who do not have counseling skill and a certain degree of health knowledge.

How extensive then should this knowledge of the health counselor be regarding mental and emotional illnesses? Reference to the role of the teacher in vision screening is again pertinent. Just as the teacher may suspect eye strain by observation and may discover defective vision by the Snellen test so, in the field of emotions, he may notice by observation that the student shows evidences of strain in his social and academic adjustments. Through counseling situations, he may discover evidences of the use of escape mechanisms by the student to the point where they are dominating his life. The ability to do this will depend on the particular knowledge and skill of the individual counselor. A consideration of some of the known facts about the more common emotional abnormalities may contribute to that knowledge.

The Normal and the Abnormal

There is no thermometer for measuring emotional status. We all do act in a mature manner at times and we act in a very immature manner at other times. The degree to which our actions show maturity determines to which class we belong. This statement must be modified to fit the child or the adolescent who is still in the act of becoming mature.

All who counsel students are cognizant of the fact that adolescence is a period of instability and that what may appear to be early signs of a deep-seated psychosis may in reality be but part of the process of growing up. Seemingly serious maladjustments may be resolved into a pattern of adjusted maturity. The psychiatrist who is working in a college health service is aware of this fact, and is alert to the danger of labelling a student psychotic during this period of constant change. Dr. Clement Fry has expressed this awareness. He states, "All but a few of the patients treated by a college mental hygiene department are so-called 'normal' boys, who react at times according to the circumstances of their lives, in much the same way as those who are popularly considered 'abnormal.' These young people have periods of anxiety and depression, they experience fears and compulsions; they are troubled by insomnia and fatigue and gastrointestinal upsets. . . . The problems which disturb them emotionally and physically arise in the normal process of their growth and in their adaptation to the special environment of a college or university." [2]

If the line between the normal and the abnormal is such a hazy one, at what point in the screening process should the counselor refer the student? There is no set answer to this question. One must consider the extent to which abnormal emotions dominate the person, because the adolescent has such varied emotional reactions to his life situation during the process of growing up. The teen-ager who dreams may be designing mental blue-prints for the homes or bridges or rocket ships of tomorrow. If he is in control of his day-dreaming and can still cope with his studies, engage in sports, and assume his share of responsibility in the social life of the school, he is merely maturing through his daydreams. As it has been so tersely stated: "He daydreams but never lets his mind fall asleep." [3] If the daydreaming takes command; if he withdraws from social contacts at school or in his community of teen-agers, if his grades begin to fall far below his mental potentialities, then he is in need of help. It is a delicate matter to decide on the point at which such help is needed. The good health counselor will sense when an interview with the student will be advantageous if the student does not voluntarily approach him. He will also sense when he is unable to give the student further help through the counseling relationship and therefore should resort to referral. In some cases, he will observe, at the first interview, that the emotional disturbance has a depth which requires immediate professional help. When this occurs, referral can be made with as much confidence as when there is a marked elevation of temperature, but the counselor may guide the student and create in him a desire for the professional help.

With these thoughts in mind, the health counselor will

[2] Clement Fry, *Mental Health in College,* New York: Commonwealth Fund, 1942, p. 4, 5.

[3] A. J. Levine, "What It Means to Be Normal," *Journal of Clinical Pathology,* Vol. IX, No. 2, p. 332, April 1948.

utilize the material presented in this chapter so that he may more intelligently cooperate with those who specialize in the field of mental health and illness.

Medical Classification of Mental Illnesses

In considering deviations from normal physical health, we are confronted with some illnesses about whose etiology very little is known. For example, in some cases of epilepsy, a causative lesion or agent has been found and a diagnosis of *symptomatic* epilepsy is made. In many cases, however, no known or specific brain disease has been found, and although scientific research is leading to a fringe of knowledge that may some day give us a clear understanding of this illness, at the present time, we diagnose the condition as *idiopathic* epilepsy. In much the same way, deviations from normal emotional and mental health may be the result of an organic lesion or agent such as arteriosclerosis of cerebral blood vessels, alcholic poisoning, or a brain tumor, and such illnesses are labelled *organic*. Other illnesses where no change in brain structure can be found are classed as *functional*.

Any classification of psychoses is misleading. Labeling a disease interferes with the ability to recognize the overlapping of symptoms. We think of it as a neat package of diagnosis, treatment, and prognosis enclosed in paper and twine that says in effect, "Now I won't need to worry about you. I know where you belong." It centers our attention on the disease entity rather than on the individual who is ill. Labeling a mental illness also tends to make us forget the physical components which are an integral part of mental disturbance. However, for the purposes of communication we need labels. When we say that one person is a psychopathic personality and another a psychoneurotic, the members of a counseling team have a common concept around which they may build their study and understanding of the individuals concerned.

As a base from which to start, we may classify emotional

and mental illnesses simply and briefly according to their known or undetermined causes, as organic, toxic, and functional conditions.

(1) **Organic psychoses.** An organic psychosis is one whose major cause is structural abnormality of brain tissue and vessels. Included in this group are senile psychosis, paresis, or psychosis resulting from injury or brain tumor.

(2) **Toxic psychoses.** The major cause of toxic psychosis is the action of a poison or toxin that may be taken into the body or produced within the body. Examples of this group are the alcoholic psychoses, the delirium of pneumonia, and psychoses due to industrial or other poisons or drugs.

(3) **Functional psychoses.** In this group belong those illnesses for which no organic defects have as yet been found, illnesses which are often considered to be learned behavior patterns. These include the various types of schizophrenia, paranoia, and manic-depressive states.

Causes of Mental Illness

Many volumes have been written about the causes of mental illness. A frank psychosis occurs when an individual has arrived at a breaking point. When a young person who withdraws from reality reaches the point where he can no longer deal with real life situations, he is classified as having schizophrenia. Preceding this point, there was a prepsychotic stage when, in most cases, signs of a near breaking point might have been noticed. Reaching back into the childhood of the individual there was a schizophrenic personality resulting from behavior patterns that were learned in infancy.

No one cause can explain any illness. We say tuberculosis is due to infection by the tuberculosis bacillus. Two college students may have been equally exposed to an active case of tuberculosis. One develops the disease; the other does not. Many factors, such as poor health habits, the lowering of normal body defenses, and emotional disturbances, may lie behind the development of tuberculosis in the first student.

In the same manner, whenever emotional symptoms predominate, there may be a crisis situation that produces the actual breaking point which results in a psychosis, but many factors, such as environment, parental rejection or overprotection, hereditary tendencies, and physical illness, are part of the background. Such factors are called predisposing causes. A *predisposing cause* of a mental illness is one which contributes to it by preparing the soil so that when an *exciting cause,* such as an emotional crisis in a life situation occurs, it can find fertile ground for the development of the psychosis. A statement of the causes of mental illness would involve a statement of the exciting causes which have been suggested in the classification of these diseases, plus a statement of all the emotional and physical disturbances during the life of the individual that have established emotional and physical patterns of behavior.

The need for objective thinking in ascertaining causes of a given case of psychosis is great. When a member of the family of a patient looks for the origin of an illness, he will always find a socially acceptable cause such as overwork with extreme fatigue, lack of vitamins, or excessive business worries. He will not admit that the ill son or brother may have experienced a lack of love and security, rejection, and frustrations because of the failure of parents and teachers to meet his emotional needs. Strecker lists a few of the childhood situations which are fraught with predisposing danger: "Failure to help children emancipate themselves from parental authority and decision however 'loving' it may be; brutal or impersonal and nonexplanatory discipline; spoiling; lack of sex information which favors maladjustment to the sexual function later in life and perpetuates sex fantasy; constant friction between parents; and many other liabilities of omission and commission on the part of parents and others entrusted with the care of children. So many of these unhygienic personal environmental factors are so directly reflected in the psychoses and psychoneuroses of adult life that we dare not discount the predisposing effect of personal environmental factors, particularly in childhood." [4]

Evidences of Abnormality

There are signs of emotional maladjustment that may point to the presence of nonpsychotic conditions, such as psychoneurosis or psychopathic personality, and signs which indicate possible prepsychotic or psychotic conditions. There are also evidences of poor emotional adjustments at the level where they may be prevented from developing into clinical illness. Excellent pamphlets designed to help teachers recognize these early signs have been prepared by government and private agencies.[5] These provide a more adequate source for information than can be given here. A brief survey of emotional abnormalities, however, may serve to provide a few basic facts which will familiarize the counselor who has limited health background with this field.

(1) **General signs of emotional maladjustment.** We have admitted that the normal and the abnormal must be differentiated by the degree rather than the kind of thoughts and actions involved in emotional responses to life situations. We are suggesting tendencies in behavior that should call attention to a possible need for counseling or referral to a medical specialist.

(a) *Shyness* that may become apparent in a number of ways. The adolescent may be overstudious, docile, and withdrawn. He may prefer seclusion and become irritable when parents or teachers attempt to break into his seclusion. He may daydream to the point where he confuses imaginative and realistic thinking.

(b) *Aggressiveness* that indicates a bullying, domineering person who is emotionally uncontrolled and antagonistic, and who is always against proposals made by other people.

[4] Edward A. Strecker, *Fundamentals of Psychiatry,* Philadelphia: J. B. Lippincott and Co., 1945, p. 14.

[5] See the bibliography of this chapter.

(c) *Strong antisocial tendencies* manifested in the overt actions of destructiveness, stealing, and lying.

(d) *Sexual deviations.*

(e) *Somatic symptoms,* such as headaches or vomiting, occurring in association with emotional disturbance.

(2) **Specific signs of emotional abnormalities.** In this section, we give a very brief description of some of the more common deviations from normal in the emotional and mental areas in both nonpsychotic and psychotic patients. We realize that the health counselor is not, as a rule, concerned with deep-seated emotional disturbances or psychoses. His contribution in such cases will be immediate referral to a psychiatrist. We also recognize the fact that psychoses cannot be understood by reading about them in a book. The understanding is possible only by the direct experience with patients which physicians, nurses, psychologists, chaplains, and social workers obtain in state or private institutions for the mentally ill. However, a brief survey may again give the health counselor needed knowledge for cooperation with the professional team.

(a) *Psychoneurosis.* This is not a psychosis. A psychoneurotic person is aware of his environment: he is oriented and can go about the daily routine of living though with dubious success. He fails, however, to adjust to his environment and to himself. It is a functional disorder rather than a disease. It is evidenced in many ways: difficulty in social adjustments, nervousness, emotional instability, oversensitiveness, fatigue, and self-centeredness. It may simulate many diseases and have somatic symptoms such as headaches, nausea, diarrhea, heart palpitation, chest pains, or tremors that may result in an erroneous diagnosis of an organic illness. It is not a temporary condition and needs referral to a specialist for determination of the deep-seated causes of the failure to adjust, and for treatment.

(b) *Hysteria.* This condition represents a form of escape from reality that is not considered psychotic. An unconscious mechanism is employed that allows the individual for the time being to avoid unbearable situations. There are such symptoms as blindness, deafness, loss of voice, loss of memory, and paralysis of arms or legs.

(c) *Psychopathic personality.* This group includes persons who have average and often superior mental ability, but whose behavior presents great problems to families and communities. They have one common characteristic: They seem to be unable to profit by experience. They show emotional instability; they do not adjust in their occupations so that they tend to have a history of frequent changes of jobs; they appear to lack a sense of ethical and moral values; they may habitually lie, steal, or cheat. These qualities are often associated with a friendly attitude, good appearance, and an excellent command of language. The result is an individual who is a danger to society. He may become an unscrupulous political boss, or may live a life in conflict with the police because of repeated minor crimes. Pathological lying and stealing with no apparent awareness of consequences or with complete disregard for them, even after repeated arrests and penalties, are typical of such a person. The condition has been considered as an integral part of the individual's personality since his birth. Much research in this field is needed if we are to arrive at a clear understanding of the causes of this disorder.

(d) *Organic psychoses.* No attempt will be made to consider individually the organic psychoses such as those resulting from arteriosclerosis of cerebral blood vessels, syphilis of the central nervous system, or damage from injury or tumor. There are some characteristics that are common to all of these types of organic disturbance. The psychosis results from temporary pressure on or permanent destruction of brain tissue that may involve the whole brain or any part of it. The specific symptoms will vary with the extent of brain damage. If the condition is not amenable to treatment, the result is a progressive deterioration. This is apparent in a lowering of mental capacity in which memory, judgment, and orientation are most affected. The memory loss is for recent rather than remote events. The senile psychosis patient may describe accurately her high school graduation party but is unable to say what she had for breakfast or whether or not her daughter visited her the very day of the examination. Defects of judgment become evident by the person's inability to give proper evaluations to facts or occurrences. There is also progressive disorientation. The elderly man who has this condition may not know what day or year it is; he may think he has been to a baseball game or has had a wonderful day of fishing even though he has been a patient in an institution for five months. He may wander away from home at any hour of day or night if he is not under careful supervision. The gradual deterioration may also result in emotional instability so that weeping becomes very easy. There may be marked relaxing of personal habits of cleanliness and neatness. Such signs of deterioration are even more evident in paresis which is the psychosis which results from syphilis attacking the brain tissue. In this particular type of organic disease, there are neurological signs and laboratory examinations which confirm the diagnosis.

Another type of organic disturbance that should be mentioned is that involving behavior disorders which result either from encephalitis or from head injury. Although the first is an infection of the brain and the second is a trauma, they give similar pictures in patterns of disturbance. Sometimes deterioration such as that described for senile psychosis occurs, even though the affected person is a child or adolescent. Other results are acute behavior disorders that may represent a complete reversal of the previous behavior of the child. Symptoms such as disobedience, defiance, lying, and cruelty must be suspected following a history of head injury or encephalitis.

(e) *Toxic psychoses.* Poisons or drugs may act chiefly by causing disturbance of consciousness with brief or prolonged periods of unconsciousness. They may, however, produce periods of delirium or depression. Alcoholism may be responsible for a series of psychotic episodes characterized by loss of consciousness or by tremors accompanied by auditory and visual hallucinations. It may result in increasing deterioration of brain tissue if the episodes are repeated, until the patient must become a permanent resident of an institution. Deficiency of the Vitamin B factors is usually acute in cases of alcoholism and this confuses the picture regarding the cause of symptoms. Since the alcoholic replaces food by drink, much of the time, the total picture involves that of lack of many of the basic foods.

(f) *Functional psychoses.* This group includes most of the mental illnesses that the layman thinks about when he speaks of *nervous breakdowns.* Among them are the conditions classified as (1) schizophrenia, (2) paranoia, and (3) manic-depressive psychosis.

(1) **Schizophrenia.** Every teacher, guidance counselor, and health educator, and many parents have been made aware of schizophrenia through pamphlets dealing with emotional health and prevention of emotional illness or through magazine or newspaper articles. This functional illness primarily affects young people; it has a strong tendency to recur; many cases, if untreated, tend to progress to a stage of extreme deterioration requiring years of institutional care. Frequently, the children who have conformed most perfectly to an adult's concept of social behavior or a teacher's idea of perfect pupils, who are studious, quiet, and refrain from asking bothersome questions, are the ones who develop this illness. Although there are several types of schizophrenia mentioned in textbooks on mental disease, the symptoms of all often overlap so that the classification of "schizophrenia, unclassified" is frequently resorted to in a medical diagnosis. For the purposes of this book, we are interested in a general view of this condition which is so varied in its aspects. We are interested, because health counselors are in a position to recognize early tendencies that may progress to a psychosis, at a stage when

wise action of parents, teachers, and counselors may make possible for the student a mature, rich life instead of one spent in an imagined world.

The schizophrenic patient is one who fundamentally evades contact with his environment. This is true for all persons with this illness regardless of the methods of escape they use. The individual may be merely indifferent, refusing to feel deeply, resulting in a shallowness of emotional experience which is characteristic of *simple schizophrenia.* He may have evaded reality by becoming mute or negative to the point of apparent cessation of bodily activity, or with phases of excitement accompanied by impulsive or destructive actions and hallucinations. These are characteristics of *catatonic* schizophrenia. He may have developed delusions of persecution accompanied by hallucinations resulting in *paranoid* schizophrenia. He may have become silly, showing emotional reactions that are inappropriate to the occasions. This would appear in the form of violent weeping at mention of a good dinner or a wedding, or gay laughter at the announcement of a death. There are delusions and hallucinations and increasing deterioration of mental ability, all of which constitute a type of schizophrenia termed *hebephrenic.*

Through all of these so-called types of the illness, however, runs the central thread of the patient's insistance on retreat from the outside world into a world of his own imagination which is in greater accord with his unsatisfied longings for romance or business success.

The arresting or curing of cases of this kind is a task for the psychiatrist. Although the future of the person who has had a complete breaking point is still far from a happy one, much has been done to restore, in many cases, the patient's ability to meet real life situations. An increasingly higher percentage of these patients is returning to family life and many are resuming responsibilities in their communities.

The concern of the health counselor is with the child or adolescent who may be helped in his life adjustment not to find the world so hostile that he will blank it out from his mind. The emphasis in psychiatry is on prevention, and this involves team action by all those who participate in the child's life.

The term "introvert" does not in itself imply an unfavorable characteristic. The introverts of every generation are most likely to become the research workers and students who make possible the progress of the next generation. The quiet, shy, retiring adolescent who would rather read than go to a dance does not automatically develop into a schizophrenic. He has, however, the characteristics of personality that provide the right soil for the development of this illness, and needs intelligent understanding by parents and others concerned in his development so that he will learn to balance his basic introversion by thoughts and actions that will keep him in touch with his friends and his environment. There is a stage in the development of the introverted child when he begins to daydream as a fulfilment of wishes and desires for things that are not part of his actual existence. If his real world offers no satisfactions at this time, if his creative energies find no outlets, if in his home and at school, he is told to be a good boy and keep still when he would like to experiment in ways that might be noisy or destructive, he will find that the daydreaming will become more and more pleasant and the life around him more and more disappointing. The health counselor contributes to the prevention of schizophrenia when he notices withdrawal tendencies in a high school student and, through the counseling relationship, helps the student grow toward realistic living, but real prevention comes in the early years when patterns of happy activity and social adjustments that are consistent with an introverted personality bring emotional and mental satisfactions.

(2) **Paranoia** is a mental illness that is different from either schizophrenia or manic-depressive psychosis. Either of these, as well as some of the organic psychoses, may show paranoid

symptoms, chief of which are ideas of persecution. The condition classified as paranoia, however, is one in which there is clarity of thought and action and where there are no hallucinations, but in which the person builds up a carefully systematized set of delusions of persecution. It is a rather rare mental illness, usually occurring in middle life, but having its origins in the experiences of many years preceding its appearance as an illness. Such persons may become dangerous to individuals or to society because they have come to believe that a person or a social system is trying to destroy them. Little is known about prevention or cure of this condition.

(3) **Manic-depressive psychoses.** It was stated in a previous chapter that the normal person has periods of elation and depression in the course of his daily experiences. The individual who is most prone to have such periods is the extrovert, who is always ready to talk or play or join in group activities. It is this type of personality structure that may result in manic-depressive psychosis if there is a breaking point in his emotional life. The person who cannot adjust to his life situation finds an escape. In the schizophrenic, this escape leads inward to a dream world. In the manic-depressive, the escape leads outward to an uninhibited expression of thoughts and actions. This may take the manic form or show as deep depression. In some cases, there is an almost rhythmic cycle from elation to depression and back to elation.

In a manic phase, the patient is overly active both physically and mentally. The "flight of ideas," so typical of such cases, results in the utterance of one statement after another with no apparent logical sequence. The manic person runs away from conflicts through his excessive activity, and also brings to the surface thoughts that have been long repressed. In the depressed stage there are often associated delusions of guilt. The depression may be expressed only by loss of interest in life and retarded thought or it may progress to the extent of a conviction of sin and unworthiness that makes the person appear to be submerged by woe so great that he cannot be aroused to even a fragment of hope. Such cases may eventually end in suicide if not treated.

Health counselors dealing with persons of middle age who are experiencing the change that occurs with cessation of sex gland activity will meet with evidence of extreme depression that may be part of this period of life. The vast majority of women and men go through this change with no disturbances or with only minor physical ailments that they disregard if they recognize their origin. A diseased condition, when it does occur, may take varied forms that suggest schizophrenic as well as depressive symptoms. The health counselor should recognize the need for referral to a psychiatrist in dealing with the mental illness of the menopause in women, and the corresponding change of life in men.

SUMMARY

Mental illness represents a very serious and increasingly urgent problem which will require the cooperation of society and of the individual citizen for its solution. Although care and treatment of the thousands of patients who occupy beds in our mental hospitals is essential, the real solution lies in prevention. Whenever a parent or teacher, or anyone who counsels children, adolescents, or adults, notices evidences of an individual's developing emotional trends or instabilities that are becoming a pattern in his life, or that are far greater in degree than is considered normal, this should be recognized as a need. This need may be met by the parent or teacher by careful guidance of a child into roads of thought and action that will help him grow physically, emotionally, and mentally into satisfying life experiences where there will be no need for or desire of escape. The need may also indicate a serious disturbance requiring the care of a specialist, but the counselor may have time and means to aid the individual in reaching the decision to ask for the specialist. In a few cases, the need will be of an emergency nature that will call for immediate help by a psychiatrist and subsequent hospitalization. But the greatest urgency for the health counselor is in the prevention of mental and emotional disturbances. The ability to help a child develop into a wholesome, adjusted adult instead of a psychoneurotic woman or man who brings constant unhappiness to self and to all members of the family is a great asset. The compensations for hours of patient listening and interchange of ideas are rewarding beyond measure when the counselor sees constructive development replacing tendencies toward regression and deterioration.

Bibliography

American Association of School Administrators, *Health in Schools, 20th Yearbook,* Washington, D. C.: American Association of School Administrators, 1942.

Baruch, D. W., "Mental Hygiene Counseling as a Part of Teacher Education," *Journal of Psychology,* January 1942.

Benson, C. E., and L. E. Alteneder, "Mental Hygiene in Teacher Training Institutions in the U. S.: A Survey," *Mental Hygiene,* April 1931.

Campbell, John D., *Everyday Psychiatry,* Philadelphia: J. B. Lippincott Co., 1945.

Carroll, Herbert A., *Mental Hygiene: The Dynamics of Adjustment,* New York: Prentice Hall, 1947.

Committee on Academic Education of the Group for the Advancement of Psychiatry, *The Role of Psychiatrists in Colleges and Universities,* Report No. 17, Topeka, Kansas: Group for the Advancement of Psychiatry, Sept. 1950. See especially the section on coordination of counseling services.

English, O. Spurgeon, and Stuart M. Finch, *Emotional Problems of Growing Up,* Chicago: Science Research Associates, 1951.

Frank, Lawrence K., "The Fundamental Needs of the Child," N. Y. Committee on Mental Hygiene of the State Charities Aid Association, *Mental Hygiene,* Vol. XXIII No. 3, July 1938.

Fry, Clement C., *Mental Health in College,* New York: The Commonwealth Fund, 1942.

Goldberger, I. H., and Grace T. Hallock, *Understanding Health,* New York: Ginn and Co., 1950. See especially Unit V.

Hymes, James L., Jr., *A Pound of Prevention,* How Teachers Can Meet the Emotional Needs of Young Children, New York: New York Committee on Mental Health of the State Charities Aid Association, 1947.

Hymes, James L., *Teacher Listen, The Children Speak. . . . ,* New York: New York Committee on Mental Health of the State Charities Aid Association, 1949.

Joint Committee on Health Problems in Education of the National Education Association and the American Medical Association, *Mental Hygiene in the Classroom,* Chicago: American Medical Association, 1940.

Jones, H. W., et al., *Blakiston's New Gould Medical Dictionary,* 1st Edition, Philadelphia: The Blakiston Co., 1949.

Leonard, Margaret, *Health Counseling for Girls,* New York: A. S. Barnes, 1944.

Levine, A. J., "What It Means to Be Normal," *Journal of Clinical Pathology,* Vol. IX No. 2, April 1948.

Menninger, William C., *Understanding Yourself,* Life Adjustment Series, Chicago: Science Research Associates, 1948.

Mueller, Kate H., *Counseling for Mental Health,* American Council on Education Studies, Series VI, Student Personnel Work, No. 8, Vol. XI, July 1947, Washington, D. C.: American Council on Education.

Palmer, Harold D., "Common Emotional Problems Encountered in a College Mental Hygiene Service," *Mental Hygiene,* 23, 544 (1939).

Sadler, William S., *Adolescence Problems, A Handbook for Physicians, Parents, and Teachers,* St. Louis: The C. V. Mosby Co., 1948.

Strecker, Edward, *Fundamentals of Psychiatry,* 3rd Edition, Philadelphia: J. B. Lippincott Co., 1945.

Thorman, George, *Toward Mental Health,* Public Affairs Pamphlet No. 120, New York: Public Affairs Committee, Inc., 1949.

Turner, C. E., *Personal and Community Health,* St. Louis; The C. V. Mosby Co., 1943.

Wickman, E. K., *Teachers and Behavior Problems,* New York: Commonwealth Fund, 1938.

CHAPTER XI

REFERRAL AND RESOURCES

The health counselor cannot help all of his clients—even his motivated clients—by himself. He often finds it necessary to use other professional resources. Some of the resources which provide counseling services and others which offer medical services are discussed in this chapter.

Many questions about referral have not been clearly answered. For example, whom does the counselor refer? When does he make the referral? How does he refer? How does he decide on one agency rather than another? In this problem area, as in others in counseling, we cannot wait for definite answers, for, if we do, death from old age might terminate the client's problem before we were prepared to aid him! Until we have the final answers, we must depend on the experience of good counselors to guide us.

Two extreme positions in the use of referrals are undesirable. There is, first, the insecure new counselor who finds haven from the threat of new counseling problems in quickly pushing the responsibility on another person. There are circumstances under which the counselor is obligated to his client to discuss early referral with him. These are suggested in the following section. However, in any counseling program, these are not the typical, everyday cases. Porter,[1] in

[1] E. H. Porter, Jr., An Introduction to Therapeutic Counseling, New York: Houghton Mifflin, 1950, p. 164.

a stimulating discussion of referral, argues against routine referral of every client to a medical specialist:

> These facts do not carry the implication that the non-medical therapist should be lax in his obligation to refer the client who presents a nonpsychological problem, but they do carry the implication that the counselor should not hasten to join the ranks of those who failed to be of help to the client.

Second, there is the egocentric counselor who rejects the use of other resources because referral means failure and inadequacy to him. This person's admission to the counseling profession was a mistake.

Skill in the process of referral and in the utilization of resources in a community enriches the counselor's professional capacities.

Why Referrals?

The counselor considers referral of a client and discusses it with him when he lacks the time or skill that the client's difficulties require for adequate assistance. He will refer a person whom he knows as a friend and with whom he could not, therefore, develop the warm, permissive, impartial counseling relationship. The counselor in certain institutions, as for example, a school, college, or an agency, will be restricted in the cases he is permitted to handle. The health counselor may be told that he is not permitted to deal with problems in sexual adjustment. The counselor may find that the nature or the characteristics of the client make it impossible for them to work together profitably. Some counselors cannot accept the antisocial, or discriminatory, or hostile attitudes of a client. In each of these cases, the client readily accepts referral. After discussing fully with him the reasons for it, the counselor refers the client to another well-qualified person and discontinues his counseling.

In other situations, the referral arises out of a supplemental need of the client for such services as medical treatment, orthopedic devices, or instruction in personal grooming. The counseling may continue or it may now terminate successfully with the referral representing part of the client's cure.

Referral may lead to continuation of counseling by another counselor; or to supplementary noncounseling service by another person or agency while counseling continues; or to a noncounseling service at the termination of the counseling.

How and When to Refer

Our check on the wisdom of the counselor remains unchanged even when applied to questions of referral, namely, what does referral mean to the client?

For the motivated client who shares a good counseling relationship with the counselor the desire for referral means opportunity for other desired assistance. Such a person can also accept the counselor's explanation of the limitation of his agency and can even welcome the counselor's information on referral possibilities.

For the motivated but highly insecure person, especially early in the counseling sessions, and for the unmotivated person, the counselor's suggestion of referral may represent rejection and defeat. It can destroy the chance of successful referral and, worse, it can impair the counseling relationship.

There is no substitute for the client's opportunity to explore his own need, his desire for referral, or for supplemental service. The counselee's self-exploration leads to acceptance and also paves the way for his effective use of the referral.

When counselor and counselee have decided together on referral, the counselor will ask the client for permission to send appropriate information to the receiving agency or to the individual specialist. Frequently, clients will request themselves that this is done, recognizing the time saving involved. Failure by the counselor to consult the counselee may lead to damaged counselor-client relationship when the client discovers that the agency knows all about him.

The nature of the referral form or letter will vary with the kind of the referral. The health counselor in the high school, referring a student to a community child-guidance clinic, will prepare, or will help prepare, a report based on all available data. He will be careful to separate facts, like those about health, performance, and family members, from his interpretation of these data. In contrast to such a comprehensive report, the health counselor, referring a student to a physician for a special medical examination, will submit little more than a statement on the expressed symptoms of the client that led to the referral. In small schools, this information is usually given orally.

Of course, when the counselor refers the client to the school or agency library for literature on health and other adjustment problems, he will prepare no referral history! If the client is shy and is likely to leave the library without the desired information, the counselor introduces him to the librarian personally or by note.

Stubbins and Cowett[2] recommend the following as good mechanics of referral from a vocational counseling agency to a case work agency:

> (1) He should be informed that the agency is willing to work with him.
>
> (2) The client should be informed and agree that information secured in his interviews will be given to the case work agency.
>
> (3) The client should be given a letter of referral to the case work agency. This we believe will help him feel more certain of acceptance.
>
> (4) Full and complete information should be sent to the case work agency quickly so that early appointments can be

[2] Joseph Stubbins, and Allan Cowett, *Referring to a Case Work Agency.* Paper read at the Midwest Regional Conference of Jewish Vocational Service Agencies, January 1951.

offered to the client. This will add to continuity of service and lessen hesitancy in accepting referral which can be caused by delay and tends to create a feeling of being forgotten.

Arbuckle[3] stresses the last point. He recommends that when a resistant student for whom a medical examination is indicated agrees to take such an examination, the teacher-counselor should take him directly to the health office.

Counseling Services for Referral

The health counselor utilizes first the counseling services within his own organization. If there is a psychiatrist, a clinical psychologist, or an educational-vocational guidance counselor, he will consult with one or more of them, depending on the nature of the problem.

If such services are not available in his institution, he will make referral to agencies in the community. Such agencies are the family welfare association, the child-guidance clinic, the local or state rehabilitation service, the veterans' administration, state mental hygiene department, public employment service, and agencies that specialize in the problems of the aged or of the infant, in marital problems, and those of minority groups. The counselor will want to be familiar with the names of specialists in private practice for those persons who prefer and can afford it.

One of the valuable tools of the health counselor is the directory of social agencies available in many large communities.[4] This lists every conceivable agency whose functions relate to the variegated aspects of adjustment and provides data which are helpful in selecting the agency for a referral. In smaller communities, this information is available through the local council of social agencies.

[3] Dugald S. Arbuckle, *Teacher Counseling,* Cambridge: Addison-Wesley Press, 1950.

[4] *Directory of Social Agencies of the City of New York,* Welfare Council of New York City, New York: Columbia University Press.

Counseling Literature

The health counselor is asked by clients for sources of information. In recent years, literature on topics that are meaningful to adolescents has been written interestingly and at the reading level of this age group. Boys and girls do not find these readings tedious and they use their contents in group discussions as well as in interviews.

Outstanding examples of such literature are the *Life Adjustment Booklets*[5] which include titles like the following:

Dating Days
Getting Along with Brothers and Sisters
Growing Up Socially
How to Live with Parents
Looking Ahead to Marriage
Understanding Sex
Understanding Yourself
You and Your Health
You and Your Mental Abilities
Your Heredity

Some books in related areas are:

Crow, Alice, and Lester Crow, *Learning to Live with Others,* Boston: D. C. Heath and Co., 1944.

Fields, Morey R., Jacob A. Goldberg, and Holger F. Kilander, *Youth Grows into Adulthood,* New York: Chartwell House, Inc., 1950.

Geisel, John B., *Personal Problems,* Francis T. Spaulding (Editor), New York: Houghton Mifflin Co., 1949.

Landis, Paul, *Your Marriage and Family Living,* New York: McGraw-Hill Book Co., 1946.

Lawton, George, *How to Be Happy though Young,* New York: The Vanguard Press, 1949.

Warters, Jane, *Achieving Maturity,* New York: McGraw-Hill Book Co., 1949.

[5] *Life Adjustment Series,* Chicago: Science Research Associates.

The publisher of the Life Adjustment Series has recently introduced a new series, the *Better Living Booklets,* designed to help parents, teachers, and others in working with children. Among the first titles are:

How to Live with Children
Self-Understanding, A First Step to Understanding Children

Health Services for Referral

The agencies and persons to whom clients may be referred for health purposes are so numerous that only a limited list will be given in outline form.

(A) In a school situation:

(1) The health service physician or nurse, if such is available. Referral for emergency medical care; for examination when an abnormal condition is suspected; for advice concerning health problems that are beyond the scope of the counselor's knowledge. The school physician will refer to outside clinics or to the family physician.

(2) The health education teacher for help regarding health habits and practices.

(3) The school dentist if one is available.

(4) The dietitian or home-economics teacher for help with nutrition problems.

(5) The professional guidance counselor for general help in counseling, and where health and guidance problems overlap.

(B) The family physician:

(1) Where there is a school physician, he will make the referral to the family physician.

(2) When the health counselor must make direct referral to a medical specialist, he should ask the client if he has a family physician. If he does, the counselor should refer the client to this physician and allow him to make referral to

other medical specialists according to his judgment. This will also apply to the family dentist.

(C) Hospital:

The nearest community or county hospital should be used. If the client has no family physician, the hospital clinics will give diagnostic and treatment services, prenatal care, child welfare care, etc.

(D) Health centers:

These are under the local board of health in larger cities. The one nearest the client should be selected. In rural areas, these centers are maintained on the county or on the state level. Mental hygiene clinics belong to this class as many of these are maintained by the state in connection with the state mental hospitals.

(E) Private agencies:

These will vary greatly with the size of the community. They will include groups which offer special services.

(1) V.N.A., Visiting Nurse Association.

When the health problem indicates the need for nursing care in the home, this agency is excellent. The service is not limited to lower income groups; it may be obtained for a moderate fee by any family in the community.

(2) Community agencies interested in family problems, such as the family welfare service, the children's aid society, the travelers' aid society where the problem involves other communities, etc.

(3) Agencies interested in specific diseases or conditions. The county tuberculosis and health association; the local or county chapter of the American Cancer Society; the nearest branch of the National Foundation for Infantile Paralysis; the nearest cardiac clinic for the heart cases, or the American Heart Association; the Society for the Hard of Hearing; the National Society for the Prevention of Blindness, etc.

(4) Agencies maintained by religious groups that offer health services as well as social services.

Resources for Health Information and Literature

Many public and private agencies provide free or low-cost material. When writing for information, it is advisable to specify your need, such as the age group for which the information will be used, or any special group, such as a foreign-speaking one. The following list is a limited one, but will suggest the types of agencies that may be contacted.

(1) Government agencies:
Federal Security Agency, Washington 25, D. C.
U. S. Children's Bureau
U. S. Public Health Service
Health Department (City)
Health Department (State)
Superintendent of Documents, Government Printing Office, Washington 25, D. C.
U. S. Department of Agriculture, Washington 25, D. C.

(2) Professional Agencies:
American Academy of Pediatrics, Inc., 636 Church Street, Evanston, Ill.
American Association for Health, Physical Education, and Recreation, 1201 16th Street, N. W., Washington 6, D. C.
American Medical Association, 535 N. Dearborn Street, Chicago 10, Ill.
American Public Health Association, 1790 Broadway, New York 19, N. Y.
National Dental Hygiene Association, 934 Shoreham Bldg., Washington 6, D. C.
National Education Association and American Medical Association Joint Committee on Health Problems in Education, 525 W. 120th Street, New York, N. Y.
National Recreation Association, 315 Fourth Avenue, New York 10, N. Y.

(3) Voluntary Agencies:

Allied Youth, Inc., 1709 M Street, N. W., Washington 6, D. C.

American Cancer Society, 47 Beaver Street, New York 4, N. Y.

American Foundation for the Blind, 15 West 16th Street, New York 11, N. Y.

American Heart Association, Inc., 1775 Broadway, New York 19, N. Y.

American Institute of Family Relations, 5287 Sunset Boulevard, Los Angeles 27, Calif.

American Social Hygiene Association, 1790 Broadway, New York 19, N. Y.

American Society for the Hard of Hearing, 1537 35th Street, N. W., Washington, D. C.

Association for Family Living, 28 E. Jackson Boulevard, Chicago 4, Ill.

Cleveland Health Museum, 8911 Euclid Avenue, Cleveland 6, Ohio

Commonwealth Fund, 41 E. 57th Street, New York 22, N. Y.

Interstate Narcotic Association, P. O. Box 1725, Paterson, N. J.

National Association to Control Epilepsy, 22 E. 67th Street, New York 21, N. Y.

National Committee for Mental Hygiene, Inc., 1790 Broadway, New York 19, N. Y.

National Foundation for Infantile Paralysis, Inc., 120 Broadway, New York 5, N. Y.

National Health Council, 1790 Broadway, New York 19, N. Y.

National Safety Council, 20 N. Wacker Drive, Chicago 6, Ill.

National Society for Crippled Children and Adults, Inc., 11 S. LaSalle Street, Chicago 3, Ill.

National Society for the Prevention of Blindness, Inc., 1790 Broadway, New York 19, N. Y.

National Tuberculosis Association, 1790 Broadway, New York 19, N. Y.

Planned Parenthood Federation of America, Inc., 501 Madison Avenue, New York 22, N. Y.

Quarterly Journal of Studies on Alcohol, 52 Hillhouse Avenue, Yale Station, New Haven, Conn.

(4) Business Groups:

Bristol-Myers Co., Educational Service Dept., 630 Fifth Avenue, New York 20, N. Y.

Good Teeth Council for Children, 17th Floor, Wrigley Bldg., 400 N. Michigan Avenue, Chicago 11, Ill.

Metropolitan Life Insurance Co., 1 Madison Avenue, New York 10, N. Y.

National Dairy Council, 111 N. Canal Street, Chicago 6, Ill.

National Live Stock and Meat Board, Department of Nutrition, 407 S. Dearborn Street, Room 825, Chicago, Ill.

Public Affairs Committee, Inc., 22 E. 38th Street, New York 16, N. Y.

Society for Visual Education, Inc., 100 E. Ohio Street, Chicago 11, Ill.

Tampax Inc., 155 E. 44th Street, New York 17, N. Y.

(5) Films:

The following may serve as a guide in obtaining current lists of films:

Directory of *U. S. Government Films* (free) U. S. Office of Education, Washington, D. C.

Encyclopaedia Britannica Films, 20 N. Wacker Drive, Chicago, Ill.

National Health Council, 1790 Broadway, New York 19, N. Y.

The names of the agencies given are, in general, those of the national organizations. The health counselor in a given community can ascertain through his local board of health the location of the nearest branch office. If this is not possible, he can write to the national office who will then notify him which is the branch nearest his own community.

Chapter XII

THE ETHICS OF HEALTH COUNSELING

The term "ethics" is a much misunderstood one in the field of medicine and health. In answer to the question, "What does medical ethics mean?" we have received such responses as:

> Jealousy between doctors makes it improper to change your doctor during an illness.
>
> My doctor can't take patients to the hospital I like because he is not on the staff there.
>
> Doctors like to protect their interests by calling them ethics.

All of these responses imply that ethics, as used in the practice of medicine, is an external affair, a system of living up to an external code by doctors and nurses that has been built up in order to give professional prestige and even coverage against criticism. They also indicate a confusion of terms which is rather common; they confuse ethics and etiquette.

In the dictionary, etiquette is defined as "the usages of polite society or professional intercourse." [1] This means doing the right thing at the right time. Professional etiquette

[1] *New Standard College Dictionary,* New York: Funk and Wagnalls Co., 1947.

in the field of medicine has undergone many changes through the years because it does involve external behavior. Especially in the early part of this century, a great concern developed for the external manifestations of professional etiquette. This became evident in the relationship between physicians and nurses, which was based on the assumption that nursing was the hand-maid of medicine. A nurse could not pass through a doorway before a physician; she had to stand in his presence even when he was seated writing orders for her; a student nurse was not allowed to attend social functions with an interne. Today, nursing has grown to the full stature of a profession, and a nurse is considered a coworker on a professional team. Professional etiquette still exists, but it is sloughing off increasingly the superficial aspects and it is accepting the definition of Emerson who described manners as "the happy way of doing things."

What then of ethics? Ethics is correctly defined as the "basic principles of right action"; it goes far deeper than the correct way of doing things. All human behavior becomes concerned with ethics, and a system of ethics develops as any group attempts to improve or standardize the individual or social behavior of its members. This applies to the medical profession and to all other professions whose members counsel with persons about health problems. It applies equally to health counselors.

The concern with "basic principles of right action" in the medical field has been present for thousands of years. One of the earliest written documents that we have is the so-called "Oath of Hippocrates." It is in reality a statement of professional ethics attributed to Hippocrates who was practicing the art of medicine around 300 B.C. His code of ethics was so practical and so lofty in its essence that it is still the accepted standard for physician-patient relationships, and adherence to the oath is declared by all those graduating from a school of medicine. A review of some of the statements made by Hippocrates may clarify our thinking regarding the ethics that constitutes the basic principles of action for the health counselor.

> I will follow the system of regimen which according to my ability and judgment I consider for the benefit of my patients and abstain from whatever is deleterious and mischievous. . . . Into whatever houses I enter I will go into them for the benefit of the sick and will abstain from every voluntary act of mischief and corruption. . . . Whatever in connection with my professional practice or not in connection with it I see or hear in the life of men which ought not to be spoken of abroad I will not divulge, as reckoning that all such should be kept secret.

"For the benefit of my patient!" The health counselor who is client-centered in his counseling relationships can qualify as an adherent to this famous oath. The counselor who uses the counseling relationship as a means of gratifying his desire for power over another human being is violating the code. The teacher in the school who accepts counseling responsibilities in the hope that this will further her chances of promotion with an increase in salary is violating a principle of right action. The social worker who gets personal satisfaction from listening to the ills and wrong-doings of others and perhaps shares with friends who are like-minded "her latest story" is not following the ethical code. The basic principle of right action for the health counselor is this principle of action "for the benefit of the client." It applies whether the client is a student in the classroom, a patient in the physician's office or hospital clinic, a parishioner in the clergyman's study, or a woman in her home who is visited by a public-health nurse or social worker.

The client comes to the counselor because he has confidence in him. He feels the need for information, for advice, for someone with whom he may discuss his problems. This may involve the revelation of thoughts and acts that are not socially acceptable. "Whatever I see or hear in the life of men which ought not to be spoken of abroad I will not divulge!" Professional ethics requires that the health counselor shall have sealed lips. The remarks of the client may provide excellent topic for conversation at a party, or even humor when told in confidence to a best friend, but those remarks belong to the client who has implicit faith in the counselor's loyalty to him. The health counselor should not betray that trust.

Professional ethics also has specific implications for the health counselor. The most important of these is that which has just been stressed: the recognition of the confidential nature of the interview. A second implication is the character of the relationship between the counselor and professional personnel or agencies in at least three types of situations:

(1) When the counselor needs information concerning the health status or economic background of the client, he should obtain this information on a professional basis. A conference with the nurse or social worker or a letter explaining that the information is needed for a counseling situation will usually bring results if there is evidence that the student or client is willing to have such information divulged. Reports that are confidential in nature cannot be given out by a medical office or social agency without the consent of the client involved. Failure to obtain such consent from the client has often resulted in the remark by a teacher that "she couldn't get any information from the health service."

(2) When a referral becomes necessary, the counselor should make the referral in writing. In some cases, such as referral of a student by a classroom teacher to the professional counselor in the school, the student himself can make the necessary appointment, but the teacher should send a brief note requesting the help of the professional person. If the referral is to an outside agency, the letter of referral should, with the consent of the client, give some details about the client as well as the reason for referral.

(3) When a referral has been made, the health counselor should no longer remain in the center of the situation. He may still show understanding and interest if he happens to see the client frequently in school or other activity, but he should not continue counseling sessions or probe into the progress of the client. It is hard for some counselors to let clients go beyond the circle of their influence, with the result that the newly established relationship is hampered in its aim to help the client grow beyond his present confusion. When a health counselor is in reality a member of a team, information concerning progress of the referred client will be given him through professional channels. If the team does not exist, then the health counselor must let knowledge of the progress of the case come from the client himself who, by his behavior and attitudes, may show increasing emotional adjustment.

The test of good counseling ethics is in its fruits. Counseling is built on a warm relationship and good communication between the counselor and client. Whatever furthers this relationship is ethical. Any act on the part of the counselor that impairs the good counseling relationship, such as betrayal of confidence or refusal to refer because of professional rivalry, is unethical.

This empirical testing of ethical practice may be carried farther by always keeping in mind the interest and possible reactions of the client. When confronted with alternative courses of action, we can decide by answering these questions: What effect will these acts have on the client? What will each course of action mean to him? Those acts that will further the positive counseling relationship and thus the client-centered goals of counseling are *ipso facto* ethical. Acts that are contrary to good counseling, and that are wilfully committed despite that known distinction are unethical.

Among the multifarious problems that may arise in counseling, many invoke ethical issues. The counselor, like other professional workers, wants to be prepared to make correct and ethical decisions. For him, this is but another aspect of his training. He cannot anticipate the varied ethical questions that will arise, but he wants to learn the principles and profit from the experience of others to face them squarely. He wants to share the thinking of others in his own and related fields and to test his ethical standards against their experience.

For this purpose, the American Psychological Association has taken an historic step in seeking to establish a code of ethical standards in clinical and consulting relationships. The Committee on Ethical Standards[2] submitted a tentative formulation of these criteria in the first of a series of fine articles. In the typically democratic manner in which it operated, the Committee went to the membership of the Association for the incidents that suggested ethical problems, and asked the psychologists, on publication of the first article, for criticisms of this draft.

We are repeating here the principles tentatively formulated, because we believe they apply to the health counselor as much as to the psychologist. We follow each principle with one or two concrete problems from the field of health counseling and allow the reader to decide for himself which is the ethical choice.

Principle 1: *The psychologist is primarily responsible to his client and ultimately to society; these basic loyalties must guide all his professional endeavors.*

Applications:

(1) Jim, age 16, has been seeing the health counselor about his acne. They have a good counseling relationship and Jim, a shy, withdrawn boy, has started to join clubs and go to parties. Jim's mother visits the counselor and asks him to influence Jim against going with "the fast gang" of boys and girls, all of whom are Jim's classmates.

(2) Bill, a good athlete and a good student, has talked

[2] APA Committee on Ethical Standards for Psychology, "Ethical Standards in Clinical and Consulting Relationships," Part I, *The American Psychologist*, 6, No. 2, 58 (1951).

with the counselor about being tired. After a thorough physical examination by his physician, which was negative, Bill realized in talking with the counselor that he had just been doing too much. He decided to drop varsity sports because he did not want to decrease his studying and reading and he could not give up his part-time job. The coach asked the counselor to persuade Bill to reconsider "for the sake of the school."

Principle 2: *The psychologist in clinical and consulting practice, mindful of the significance of his work in the lives of other people, must strive at all times to maintain highest standards of excellence, valuing competence and integrity more than expedience or temporary success.*

Applications:

(1) The manager in a public employment office tells the counselor handling the handicapped job applicants to "get tough with them. We're babying them too much and they're holding off until they get the jobs they want. We've got to get more handicapped applicants placed."

(2) The nurse-counselor was interviewing an anxious mother who was concerned about the illness of her child. The mother asked if she would repeat what she had said about the baby's diet. The counselor replied, "Madam, we're very busy here, and I can't be repeating things. You'd better listen carefully."

Principle 3: *The psychologist in clinical or consulting practice should refuse to suggest, support, or condone any undertaking involving unwarranted assumptions, invalid applications or unjustified conclusions in the use of psychological instruments or techniques.*

Application:

Mary does very poorly in her sixth grade class. The principal asks the health counselor to interview her and decide if she is feeble-minded.

Principle 4: *Individuals and agencies in clinical and consulting practice are obligated to define for themselves the nature and directions of their loyalties and responsibilities in any particular undertaking, to inform all involved of these commitments, and to carry them out conscientiously.*

Application:

The counselor in the school of nursing has been counseling a student nurse. The student has discussed many intimate details of her past and has asked the counselor not to disclose these. The supervisor of nursing education asks the counselor to show her the interim notes so that she can better understand the student.

Principle 5: *It is unethical for a psychologist to offer services outside his area of training and experience or beyond his level of competence.*

Applications:

(1) During the course of an interview, involving the client's feelings about her complexion, the counselor advised her to buy a sun-ray lamp to use in daily treatments, and to take vitamins.

(2) The client reported that he suffered from headaches every time he had an exam. The counselor told him it was psychological and to stop worrying.

These ethical standards constitute a modern implementation of the Hippocratic Oath.

Chapter XIII

THE EVALUATION OF COUNSELING

Counselors want to increase their counseling proficiency. They want to develop their professional ability in order to be of maximum service to their clients. The counselor who maintains an interest in growth should have no fear of stagnation, and if he is concerned with the effectiveness of his work, he should have no doubt about his contributions to his clients.

Growth means change and change means giving up the old for the new. Great thinkers in the field of counseling and other therapy have not hesitated to discard their earlier concepts for newer ones, even when their names were closely linked with these concepts. Some followers of Freud failed to keep up with revisions in his concepts of the therapist-patient relationship, just as today some of Rogers' followers have failed to keep pace with the changes between 1942 and 1951 in his thinking about the counselor-client relationship. These revisions were a result of careful examination of the process of counseling, of the attitudes of counselor and client, and of the outcomes of the counseling in terms of changes in personality and in behavior.

Evaluation means appraisal of one's work in achieving the goals one has set for one's counseling. Evaluation cannot be made unless the counselor has the strength to admit to imperfections and errors and to analyze his own work with some degree of self-detachment and objectivity. The absence of these qualities for evaluation points to an individual of professional mediocrity.

A first step in evaluation is in determining the criteria of good counseling. What are the goals I set for myself?, the counselor asks himself. To what degree have I achieved these goals?

Criteria of Good Counseling

Discussions on the criteria of good counseling frequently lead to the injection of the counselor's personal values. Good counseling then becomes the process that leads to behavior patterns which the *counselor* regards as desirable. There is then the danger that the process will be examined for its success in leading people to accept the counselor's values, as for example, abstinence, eating a balanced diet, attending church, avoidance of premarital sexual relations, and the daily practice of calisthenics. There is the equal danger that another counselor will look for these evidences of success: flexibility in the use of liquor, indifference to a balanced diet, rejection of religious practices, freedom in premarital relations, and the avoidance of exercise. These dangers can be avoided only by judging the counseling in terms of its success in guiding the client to meet his needs as *he* experiences them.

We propose as the primary criterion of successful counseling the changes in the client's self-perception in the direction of greater harmony with the realities of his experience. The client can then achieve more effective living, by which we mean the clarification of his goals in the light of better understood reality, and the activation of a design for their attainment. This primary criterion applies equally to the motivated client in the counseling interview and the unmotivated subject of the counselor's case-work activities.

The "ultimate goals on counseling" suggested by Robinson[1] are akin to ours except that they are seen from the counselor's perspective rather than the client's:

> Since clients are usually unhappy with their present adjustment, it is obvious that counselors should seek to increase the client's feelings of well-being and adjustment. Counseling success can in part be evaluated in these terms (page 16).
>
> Effective counseling should also result in the disappearance of symptoms of maladjustment. The mere inhibition of symptoms of maladjustment is of little value, but with an underlying improvement in adjustment these symptoms should disappear or at least decrease (pages 16-17).
>
> Finally, effective counseling should result in better adjustment of the client to his environment and to society (page 17).
>
> In brief, then, the goals of counseling are to increase a client's feeling of personal adjustment and his actual effectiveness in society—not only in immediate but also in later situations (page 20).

What is "better adjustment"? Some studies have made improved grades, or increased participation in extracurricular activities, or greater earnings—one year after counseling—the criteria of adjustment. Yet for some persons these could be evidences of maladjustment. Conceivably, for one person, more organized living, more sleep and greater regularity in eating could be evidences of better adjustment, while for another—for a person who has been plagued by rigidity in his pattern of living, thinking, and feeling—the very opposite would indicate better adjustment. There is no sounder criterion than a change in personal meanings that permits self-enhancement through one's experience of reality.

Establishing a criterion is largely academic until it can be applied to the rigorous tasks of evaluation. How are we to

[1] Francis P. Robinson, *Principles and Procedures in Student Counseling*, New York: Harper and Bros., 1950.

determine that meanings have been changed and that the change has been in the direction of the realities of experience? There is still no completely satisfactory answer to this question. Yet, we are making impressive progress in our ability to analyze, understand, and evaluate counseling success. The research of the past decade has been extremely heartening. We have learned to apply the principles of research to the interpersonal counseling relationship which had once been regarded as too fragile for the heavy hands of science.

We propose as a secondary criterion the extent to which the counselor's practices in the counseling interview conform to desirable practices in counseling. By desirable practices we mean those which have tentatively been so established by research and also those which—although not yet tested by research—are consistent with the counselor's understanding of behavior and the dynamics of the counseling relationship. This is an important criterion because it focuses on the counselor himself and because it is more practicable for the busy counselor than the more complex study of counseling outcomes.

Research on Evaluation

The numerous studies on counseling effectiveness cut across all areas of adjustment. Although we are interested in learning how to evaluate counseling in the health area, we can draw on the experience of persons in other special counseling fields.

The breadth of evaluative studies in the field of guidance is seen in Froehlich's[2] review of the literature published during the period of 1921 to 1947. He classified the studies taken from one hundred and seventy-seven sources into seven categories, according to the method used in the investigation, and made a critical analysis of each method.

[2] C. P. Froehlich, *Evaluating Guidance Procedures, A Review of the Literature,* Washington, D. C.: Federal Security Agency, Office of Education, Miscellaneous No. 3310, 1949.

In an ambitious study of guidance practices in secondary schools, Kefauver and Hand[3] found serious shortcomings, particularly in the value of the group guidance procedures examined. This study has itself been criticized for weaknesses in the methodology of evaluation. A contribution from the investigation pertinent to health counseling is the judgment of three hundred and forty-five specialists, including principals, counselors, and professors of guidance and of secondary education, on the importance of various "health guidance objectives."

Health Guidance Objectives of Great Importance

(1) To contribute to the effectiveness of the educational program of the school in preparing students for healthful living

(2) To define and to reduce the extent of remediable health defects

(3) To lead students to plan a well-balanced program of physical activities

(4) To lead students to plan and to carry out a program of preparation for healthful living

(5) To help students inform themselves about the importance of health and the need for health education

(6) To help students determine their physical strengths, weaknesses, and needs

Health Guidance Objectives of Moderate Importance

(7) To help students inform themselves about the subjects and activities which contribute to sound health

(8) To help students inform themselves about the health services, clinics, etc., of the school and of the community

(9) To lead former students to have a continuous plan of activity and study to prepare for more healthful living

[3] Grayson Kefauver and Harold C. Hand, *Appraising Guidance in Secondary Schools,* New York: The Macmillan Co., 1941, pp. 30-31.

In another critical review of evaluative techniques in guidance, Travers[4] stated that the guidance interview is a learning situation and he proposed that counselors employ the evaluative techniques used in education.

> In organized learning situations in education, goals are established, procedures are developed for attaining those goals, and methods are devised for determining the extent to which the goals are achieved.

The goal of the counseling interview, as we picture it, is to establish the conditions in which the client can evaluate *his own goals* and to prepare to achieve them.

Snyder's[5] report on the status of psychotherapeutic counseling includes a review of evaluating articles for each of the different counseling approaches. One of the trends that he commends:

> . . . is the tendency to recognize that there is no method that cannot be subjected to scientific examination. Even the most systematized of theoretical constructs are now being explored. Many writers are no longer satisfied to present only case histories without some objectification of measurement of outcome. Psychotherapy, while long an art, is in the early stages of becoming a science.[6]

He concludes that the phonographically recorded interview is the most significant experimental contribution to psychotherapy.

Two critical analyses of evaluative studies in the group work area are: Hoppock's[7] on the effectiveness of group guid-

[4] R. M. W. Travers, "A Critical Review of Techniques Evaluating Guidance," *Educational and Psychological Measurement,* 9, 211 (1949).

[5] W. U. Snyder, "The Present Status of Psychotherapeutic Counseling," *Psychological Bulletin,* 44, 297 (1947).

[6] W. U. Snyder, "The Present Status of Psychotherapeutic Counseling," *Psychological Bulletin,* 44, 368 (1947).

[7] Robert Hoppock, *Group Guidance, Principles, Techniques, and Evaluation,* New York: McGraw Hill, 1949, Part III.

ance practices in high schools and colleges and Zlatchin's[8] on group therapy.

Many investigations have provided us with evaluative procedures, such as those for the appraisal of student personnel programs,[9,10] and those for measuring and analyzing the counseling process.[11,12,13]

Among the numerous studies on the outcome of counseling, there have been several evaluations of college counseling programs.[14,15] They also include the rich yield of research findings on nondirective counseling. These are synthesized by Rogers[16] in his discussion on changes in personality and changes in behavior produced by client-centered counseling. Before quoting Rogers' summary of these findings, we must add both his and our own words of caution.

Few persons now in health counseling engage in the complete process of counseling evaluated in the studies reported by Rogers. Some of the health counselor's clients need this kind of aid, but the counselor lacks the time, or the skill, or both. When professional specialists are available, clients such as these are referred by the health counselor; otherwise they go unaided. Nevertheless, these evaluative studies indicate

[8] Philip J. Zlatchin, *The Effects of Group Therapy upon Some Aspects of Behavior, Social Relationships, and Personal Attitudes of Adolescent Problem Boys,* unpublished Ph.D. thesis, New York University, 1950.

[9] Frances M. Wilson, *Procedures in Evaluating a Guidance Program,* New York: Bureau of Publication, Teachers College, Columbia University, 1945.

[10] C. Gilbert Wrenn and Robert B. Kamm, "A Procedure for Evaluating a Student Personnel Program," *School and Society,* 67, 266 (1948).

[11] E. H. Porter, Jr., "The Development and Evaluation of a Measure of Counseling Interview Procedures," I. The Development, II. The Evaluation, *Educational and Psychological Measurement,* 3, 105, 215 (1943).

[12] Julius Seeman, "A Study of the Process of Nondirective Therapy," *Journal of Consulting Psychology,* 13, 157 (1943).

[13] Nathaniel J. Raskin, *An Objective Study of the Locus of Evaluation Factor in Psychotherapy,* Ph.D. thesis, University of Chicago, 1949.

[14] Barbara A. Kirchheimer, David W. Axelrod, and George X. Hickerson, Jr., "An Objective Evaluation of Counseling," *Journal of Applied Psychology,* 33, 249 (1949).

[15] J. R. Toven, "Appraising a Counseling Program at the College Level," Occupations, 23, 459 (1945).

[16] Carl R. Rogers, *Client-Centered Therapy,* New York: Houghton Mifflin, 1951.

the therapeutic power of the kind of counseling relationship we have described; and they suggest the quality of service that will be available when much needed additional staff members, trained in counseling, will have been added to our schools, colleges, child guidance clinics, health agencies, and other institutions.

Rogers cautions, first, that the personality tests used to measure change in personality "are themselves of dubious validity," and second, that the "modest but important" personality changes that occurred did not make the clients unrecognizably different from what they had been:

> Do the changes which occur in client-centered therapy alter the basic structure of personality? The studies which have been cited would seem to justify an answer along these lines. When an investigation is made of a randomly selected group of clients receiving client-centered therapy, it is generally found that one outcome of the experience is a significant degree of change in the basic personality configuration. This change appears to be in the direction of: an increased unification and integration of personality; a lessened degree of neurotic tendency; a decreased amount of anxiety; a greater degree of acceptance of self and of emotionality as a part of self; increased objectivity in dealing with reality; more effective mechanisms for dealing with stress-creating situations; more constructive feelings and attitudes; and a more effective intellectual functioning. On the basis of limited evidence, it would appear that these personality changes are relatively permanent, often continuing in the directions already described.
>
> Does the process of client-centered therapy involve any change in the behavior and actions of the client? Pulling together the threads from these various studies, we may say that, during the process of client-centered therapy, the evidence at present available suggests that the client's behavior changes in these ways: He considers, and reports putting into effect, behavior which is more mature, self-directing, and responsible than the behavior he has shown heretofore; his

> behavior becomes less defensive, more firmly based on an objective view of self and reality; his behavior shows a decreasing amount of psychological tension; he tends to make a more comfortable and effective adjustment to school and to job; he meets new stress situations with an increased degree of inner calm, a calm which is reflected in less psychological upset and more rapid psychological recovery from these frustrating situations than would have been true if they had occurred prior to therapy.[17]

Practical Methods of Evaluation

These are impressive studies, you will say, and I am glad I am familiar with them, but what can I do to evaluate my own counseling? What does a part-time school counselor with a heavy load of classes and cases do? Or, an instructor in a school of nursing who has time for counseling, but no time nor skill for scientific research? Or, the YMCA secretary, the community-center group leader, the pastor, each one wishing to add counseling to his many other duties? Will they have to discard any plans for professional growth through evaluation if this entails the complexities of the reported investigation? We shall attempt to answer these questions in the remainder of this chapter.

The most important element for success in counseling is the counselor. He can evaluate his effectiveness by examining the nature of the relationship that he creates with the client. Appel,[18] a psychiatrist, wrote:

> No therapy, however helpful and useful in itself, will be of value unless a constructive relationship is developed between patient and doctor. . . . He should enable the patient to feel that he, the therapist, has real interest in him and his problems.

[17] Carl R. Rogers, *Client-Centered Therapy,* New York: Houghton Mifflin, 1951, page 186.

[18] Kenneth E. Appel, "Psychiatric Therapy," in J. McV. Hunt's *Personality and the Behavior Disorders,* New York: Ronald Press Co., 1944, p. 1157.

In a recent summary of the findings of evaluative studies of guidance, Blum and Balinsky[19] stress the importance of warmth in counseling.

Reporting on a study of ratings given by supervisors to seventy-five beginning counselors in three hundred and seventy interviews, Robinson[20] says:

> Beginning counselors' biggest difficulty seems to be a tendency to take too much responsibility. Note the high votes for "not giving the Client responsibility," "talk too much," "too many questions," "judicial, authoritarian" and "counselor structures too much." This tendency is in agreement with Sherman's finding that the average responsibility division of expert counselors was better than that for inexperienced counselors. . . . Part of this is due to a lack of understanding of how the counselor and client work together as a team. But in part it is also sometimes due to the feeling of personal involvement which many beginning counselors have in their counseling, i.e., they feel that it will be a reflection on their ability if they do not produce results and so they work too hard at it.

Carnes and Robinson[21] studied the relationship between the amount of talking by the client in the counseling interview and the effectiveness of the interview. Interview effectiveness was inferred from (1) growth in counselee insight into his problems, (2) quality of the working relationship between counselor and counselee, as evidenced by counselee resistance or indifference, and (3) client responsibility for the progress of the interview. The investigators found that there was a positive relationship, though a low one, between the amount of counselee talk and his insight

[19] Milton L. Blum, and Benjamin Balinsky, *Counseling and Psychology*, New York: Prentice-Hall, 1951.

[20] Francis P. Robinson, *Principles and Procedures in Student Counseling*, New York: Harper and Bros., 1950, p. 158.

[21] Earl F. Carnes and Francis P. Robinson, "The Role of Client Talk in the Counseling Interview" in Arthur H. Brayfield's *Readings in Modern Methods of Counseling*, New York: Appleton-Century-Crofts, 1950, p. 414.

and between counselee talk and working relationship. There was a higher relationship between counselee talk and counselee responsibility for the progress of the interview.

These studies and the independent judgment of dozens of experienced counselors define the desirable behavior of the counselor as follows: The counselor is a warm, accepting person who gains the cooperation of the client, encourages the cooperation of the client, encourages the client to express himself freely and to assume responsibility for the progress of the interview. Fiedler's studies[22] have now given us the first direct corroboration of the importance of this kind of relationship. His work suggests that the primary characteristic of the good counselor, the characteristic that differentiates the expert from the nonexpert, is his ability to communicate with the client. To achieve this, the good counselor maintains rapport; he follows and understands the client and respects him as an equal.

The studies have given us a criterion of good counseling, and by using it, the new counselor can evaluate his work. He should not feel discouraged at finding shortcomings, for Fiedler found that experience was the chief variable between the good and the poor counselors. Evaluation and correction are means of speeding up the process of becoming a skilled counselor.

Evaluation of the counseling relationship is best accomplished when one has tangible material to evaluate. Surely, the experienced counselor can sense the feelings of the client toward him and the atmosphere in which they operate. This is not so true for the inexperienced counselor. In any event, even the experienced counselor is restricted to the grosser aspects of the counseling relationship if he attempts evaluation without a record of the interview.

Some counselors learn to note down rapidly cue words of the client and cues to their own responses, which they com-

[22] Fred E. Fiedler, "The Concept of the Ideal Therapeutic Relationship," *Journal of Consulting Psychology*, 14, (1950).

plete after the interview. Others are more fortunate in that they have available electrical recording equipment. The declining cost of tape and wire recorders makes it feasible for institutions to provide these highly valuable instruments for their counselors.

What should the counselor look for in examining his success in creating the desirable relationship? One of the valuable by-products of Fiedler's work is a group of statements considered more characteristic of experts than nonexperts and another group less characteristic of experts than of nonexperts. These statements are taken from a total list of 75, and they are identified by the category in which they were unanimously placed by the judges in the study. (Fiedler uses the word therapist rather than counselor.)

Statements More Characteristic of Experts Than of Nonexperts

I. Communication

Communication and understanding are good

(1) The therapist is usually able to get what the patient is trying to communicate.

(2) The therapist is well able to understand the patient's feelings.

(3) The therapist really tries to understand the patient's feelings.

(4) The therapist always follows the patient's line of thought.

(5) The therapist usually catches the patient's feelings.

Communication and understanding are excellent

(1) The therapist's comments are always right in line with what the patient is trying to convey.

(2) The therapist is able to participate completely in the patient's communication.

(3) The therapist is never in any doubt about what the patient means.

(4) The therapist's tone of voice conveys the complete ability to share the patient's feelings.

II. Emotional Distance

The therapist is emotionally neutral

(1) The therapist's feelings do not seem to be swayed by the patient's remarks.

III. Status

The therapist maintains peer relationship with the patient

(1) The therapist gives and takes in the situation.

Statements Less Characteristic of Experts Than of Nonexperts

I. Communication

No communication is possible

(1) The therapist cannot maintain rapport with the patient.

(2) The therapist shows no comprehension of the feelings the patient is trying to communicate.

(3) The therapist's own needs completely interfere with his understanding of the patient.

Communication is poor

(1) The therapist often flounders around before getting the patient's meaning.

(2) The therapist often misses the point the patient is trying to get across.

(3) The therapist is unable to understand the patient on any but a purely intellectual level.

(4) The therapist finds it difficult to think along the patient's lines.

II. Emotional Distance

The therapist draws away from or rejects the patient

(1) The therapist feels disgusted by the patient.

The therapist is somewhat cool toward the patient

(1) The therapist feels somewhat tense and on edge.

(2) The therapist seems to be a little afraid of the patient.

The therapist tends to be too close, is sticky

(1) The therapist showers the patient with affection and sympathy.

III. Status

The therapist tends to look up to and defer to the patient

(1) The therapist assumes an apologetic tone of voice when commenting.[23]

For those who work without supervision, it is not a simple matter to find deficiencies in one's own counseling. We cannot always be sufficiently objective to recognize our errors. Asking another member of the staff to lend an "impartial ear" is one way of dealing with this obstacle to appraisal. A case conference with noncounselors, built around an interview recording or some other report of an interview, serves both the counselor's need for evaluation and the other staff members' need for understanding of the counseling process.

As we play back the recording of an interview, we see the effect we have on the client. We note the warmth of our expression at the beginning and the increased relaxation of the client; or the fright or chill in our voice and the continued tension of the client. We hear our genuine acceptance of his feelings or of his version of his problem, followed quickly by further expression of feeling; or we hear our disagreement with his version of his problem, followed by silence, or a monosyllabic response and growing resistance.[24] We recognize that our genuine belief in his ability to deal with his problem leads to much counselee talk, much expression of feeling, much new insight as he gains new meanings; or we recognize that our inability to accent the hypothesis that the individual has the capacity to cope with his difficulties has provoked us to interfere with the direction of the interview and has confused the client.[25] We see that when

[23] Fiedler, F. E., "A Comparison of Therapeutic Relationships . . ." *Journal of Consulting Psychology*, **14**, 438, 439 (1950).

[24] Richard Hogan, *The Development of a Measure of Client Defensiveness in a Counseling Relationship*, Ph.D. thesis, University of Chicago, 1948.

[25] Nathaniel J. Raskin, *An Objective Study of the Locus of Evaluation Factor in Psychotherapy*, Ph.D. thesis, University of Chicago, 1949.

we grant his request for information on referral, for literature, or for explanation of our respective roles in the interview, there is a forward spurt in the counseling that comes from the team-work feeling; and that when we deny his request, there are annoyance and resistance.

Having a record of the counseling interview also enables us to examine the change in client meanings that grow from the counseling relationship. Rogers summarized these changes as they were ascertained in a series of significant studies.[26] He found that the changes occur in three general ways. We are quoting these separately, and following each with questions that the counselor will want to answer to determine the growth of his client:

> He perceives himself as a more adequate person with more worth and more possibility of meeting life.[27]

(1) Has the client felt free to express negative feelings about himself?

(2) Has he been discouraged?

(3) Does he now, as the interviewing proceeds, find positive qualities in himself?

(4) Is he more hopeful about achieving satisfactions in life?

He permits more experiential data to enter awareness and

[26] Some of these studies are:

Curran, C. A., *Personality Factors in Counseling*, New York: Grune and Stratton, 1945.

Raimy, Victor C., "Self Reference in Counseling Interviews," *Journal of Consulting Psychology*, 12, 153 (1948).

Seeman, Julius, "A Study of the Process of Nondirective Therapy," *Journal of Consulting Psychology*, 13, 157 (1949).

Sheerer, Elizabeth T., "An Analysis of the Relationship between Acceptance of and Respect for Self and Acceptance of and Respect for Others in Ten Counseling Cases," *Journal of Consulting Psychology*, 13, 169 (1949).

Snyder, W. U., "An Investigation of the Nature of Nondirective Psychotherapy," *Journal of General Psychology*, 33, 193 (1945).

Stock, Dorothy, "An Investigation into the Interrelations between the Self-concept and Feelings Directed toward Other Persons and Groups," *Journal of Consulting Psychology*, 13, 176 (1949).

[28] Carl R. Rogers, *Client-Centered Therapy*, New York: Houghton Mifflin, 1951, p. 139.

thus achieves a more realistic appraisal of himself, his relationships, and his environment.[28]

(1) Does he talk more freely about subjects that were painful to him?

(2) Can he admit to deficiencies in himself that he had hidden before?

(3) Can he admit to negative attitudes of other people that he has refused to accept?

(4) Does he also recognize the positive qualities about himself and his environment that he had not perceived before?

He tends to place the basis of standards within himself, recognizing that the "goodness" or "badness" of any experience or perceptual object is not something inherent in that object, but is a value placed on it by himself.[28]

(1) Was he indecisive at the start of counseling?

(2) Was he torn between needs of his own and values at conflict with his needs?

(3) Does he develop personal strength to make judgments or values of his own?

(4) Does he become more independent and ready to decide?

Such changes in self-perception as these are brought about in the counseling interview. They come about when the desirable counseling relationship is created. These changes may serve as criteria of effective case-work, though the counselor must use external indicators of such change rather than the expressed feelings of the client in the interview. He must make inferences of changed meanings from the individual's behavior, his achievement, and his social integration.

There are great satisfactions in counseling that make evaluation and growth worth while. One of them is helping individuals deal more adequately with their problems. Another is knowing that effective counseling leads to clearer percep-

[28] Carl R. Rogers, *Client-Centered Therapy,* New York: Houghton Mifflin, 1951, p. 139.

tion and to greater objectivity. Still another is the knowledge that as clients develop greater self-respect they show greater respect for others.[29]

It is satisfyng to know that in one's professional work, one can make such contributions in a world desperately in need of objectivity and respect for others.

BIBLIOGRAPHY

Porter E. H., Jr., *An Introduction to Therapeutic Counseling,* New York: Houghton Mifflin Co., 1950, chapters 2, 8, and 9.

Robinson, Francis P., *Principles and Procedures in Student Counseling,* New York: Harper and Bros., 1950, chapters 5 and 6.

Rogers, Carl R., *Client-Centered Therapy,* New York: Houghton Mifflin Co., 1951.

[29] Dorothy Stock, "An Investigation into the Interrelations between the Self-Concept and Feelings Directed toward Other Persons and Groups," *Journal of Consulting Psychology,* 13, 176 (1949).

GLOSSARY

For meanings of medical words or terms not included in this glossary, the reader is referred to *Blakiston's New Gould Medical Dictionary;* First Edition, Philadelphia: The Blakiston Company, 1949.*

Accomodation: the ability of the eye to focus on objects at different distances.

Acne: infection of the sebaceous glands of the skin.

Addiction: a state of dependence on a drug.

Addison's disease: a disease caused by hypofunction of the adrenal cortex and characterized by pigmentation of the skin, prostration, anemia, low blood pressure, and digestive disturbance.

Adenoids: growth of lymphoid tissue in the nasopharynx.

Adrenal cortex: the outer portion of an adrenal gland.

Allergy: a condition of exaggerated sensitivity to a substance which is harmless in similar amounts for most people.

Ambivalence: simultaneous existence of contradictory emotions toward the same person or object; for example, mixed love-hate feelings.

Anemia: a condition in which the red corpuscles of the blood are deficient in hemoglobin and/or reduced in number.

Anorexia: lack of appetite for food.

Antibiosis: (adjective: antibiotic) an association between two or more organisms which is harmful to one of them.

Antibody: a substance manufactured by the body cells to neutralize the toxin of a specific kind of bacterium or virus, or to unite

* This glossary includes some terms which are not used in the text, but which may be helpful to the health counselor.

with the bacterium itself so as to make it more vulnerable to attack by phagocytes.

Anxiety neurosis: a state of anxiety caused by inner conflict.

Arteriosclerosis: the condition brought about by degenerative changes in the arteries producing thickening (hardening) of their walls.

Ascorbic acid: vitamin C.

Asthma: a spasmodic contraction of the bronchial tubes which results in difficult breathing; usually an allergic reaction.

Astigmatism: an irregularity of the refracting surfaces of the eye interfering with the sharp focusing of light rays on the retina.

Audiogram: a graphic record showing the variations of auditory acuity of an individual, as indicated by an audiometer test.

Auricle: ear-shaped structure or appendage. This term is commonly used for the external ear flap, or for the first chamber of the heart which receives the blood from the veins.

Bacillus: a rod-shaped organism.

Basal metabolic rate: the amount of energy expended per unit of time under basal conditions, that is, when the body is at complete rest. It represents the minimal amount of energy required to carry on the vital activities of the body, such as breathing and heart action.

Beri-beri: a disease of the nerves due to a lack of thiamine.

Bronchial tubes: primary branches of the trachea.

Bursitis: inflammation of a bursa, which is a sac filled with fluid and situated at a place in the tissues at which friction would otherwise develop.

Calorie: a heat unit; the amount of heat required to raise the temperature of one liter water 1°C.

Caries: decay; (dental: disease or decay of teeth.)

Cataract: partial or complete opacity of the crystalline lens of the eye.

Catharsis (mental): emotional relief obtained through the overt expression of unpleasant memories.

Cerumen: waxlike secretion within the external passage of the ear.

Cervical: pertaining to the neck; the part corresponding to the neck, e.g., the cervical part of the uterus, "cervix uteri."

Clinical: pertaining to the symptoms of a disease; relating to bedside treatment.

Comedones: blackheads found in the skin.
Conjunctivitis: inflammation of the transparent mucous membrane covering the eye and lining the eyelids.
Contusion: a bruise.
Cumulative: increasing, adding to.
Deafness: loss, lack, or impairment of the sense of hearing. Usually refers to total loss in the ear concerned.
Decibel: a unit for measuring the loudness of sounds.
Defective hearing: partial loss of sense of hearing.
Defense mechanisms: conscious or unconscious reactions designed to minimize or avoid sources of mental distress.
Delusion: a false belief; the person having delusions is unable to accept proof that they are false.
Dementia praecox: see schizophrenia.
Dermatitis: an inflammation of the skin.
Dorsum: the back. Any part corresponding to the back, as the dorsum of the hand.
Dysmenorrhea: difficult or painful menstruation.
Duodenum: the first part of the small intestine beginning at the pylorus.
Eczema: an acute or chronic noninfectious, inflammatory disease of the skin.
Edema: swelling of tissues.
Electrocardiogram: a graphic record, made by an electrocardiograph, of the electrical potential differences due to heart action; referred to as ECG.
Electroencephalogram: a graphic record made by an electroencephalograph, an instrument for recording the electrical activity of the brain; referred to as EEG.
Encephalitis: inflammation of the brain.
Endocarditis: inflammation of the inner lining of the heart.
Endocrine gland: a gland discharging its secretion directly into the blood.
Epilepsy: a disorder of the central nervous system, manifested by transient episodes of unconsciousness or psychic dysfunction with or without convulsive movements.
Epistemology: critical investigation of the nature and validity of human knowledge.
Etiology: the science or study of the causes of disease.

Eustachian tube: a canal connecting the middle ear with the pharynx.

Fibrosis: formation of fibrous tissue.

Fluoroscope: a device for examining deep tissues by means of x-rays.

Functional: denotes a disease in which no tissue damage has been demonstrated and no organic cause found to the present time.

Fungus: a plant of the mold type.

Gingivitis: inflammation of the gums.

Goiter: enlargement of the thyroid gland.

Hallucination: a sensation without an object; a condition where a patient "hears" or "sees" voices or visions that do not have a starting point or a sensory stimulus.

Hemoglobin: the oxygen-carrying substance of red blood corpuscles.

Hormone: a substance produced in one organ which is discharged into the blood and excites functional activity in another organ.

Hyperfunction: excessive function; overactivity, as of a gland.

Hyperopia: farsightedness.

Hypertension: high blood pressure.

Hypertrophy: an increase in the size of a tissue or organ independent of the general growth of the body.

Hypofunction: diminished function; underactivity, as of a gland.

Hypotension: low blood pressure.

Hysteria: lack of control over the emotions or acts.

Identification: a mental mechanism by which an individual, without conscious awareness, satisfies frustrated desires by psychologically assuming the role of another person.

Immunity: a condition of a living organism in which it resists and overcomes infection.

Impetigo: an inflammatory skin disease.

Insulin: a hormone produced in the pancreas.

Kyphosis: angular curvature of the spine; humpback.

Lesion: an alteration of structure or of functional capacity by injury or disease.

Leucocytosis: an increase in the number of white (colorless) blood corpuscles.

Leucopenia: a reduction in the number of white blood corpuscles.

Lobectomy: excision of a lobe of an organ or gland.

Lordosis: forward curvature of the spine; hollow back

Lumbar: pertaining to the lower part of the spine.

Lymph nodes: a glandular center in which lymph vessels converge.

Malaise: uneasiness, discomfort, distress.

Mastoid: the lower portion of the temporal bone of the skull, located immediately behind the ear.

Mantoux: skin test to determine presence of primary infection by tuberculosis bacillus.

Migraine headache: paroxysmal intense pain in the head; of unknown etiology.

Moron: a mentally defective adult who has not advanced beyond the mental stage of a twelve-year-old child.

Myocarditis: inflammation of the muscular tissue of the heart.

Myopia: nearsightedness.

Narcotic: any drug that produces sleep and relieves pain.

Neuritis: inflammation of a nerve.

Neurosis: see psychoneurosis.

Niacin: Nicotinic acid; antipellagra factor of vitamin B complex.

Ophthalmologist: a physician who has specialized in diseases of the eye.

Optician: a maker of optical instruments or lenses.

Optometrist: one who has made a study of the eye, especially its measurement for refractive errors.

Organic: affecting the structure of organs.

Orthopedist: a specialist in the corrective treatment of deformities and diseases of the locomotor apparatus.

Otitis media: inflammation of the middle ear.

Otologist: physician specializing in diseases and abnormalities of the ear.

Paranoia: a functional mental disorder with delusions, particularly of a persecutory type.

Parathyroid: one of the four small glands in back of the thyroid gland.

Paresis: general slight paralysis: as used in this text, it refers to *general paresis* which is a form of neurosyphilis, involving chiefly the cortex of the frontal and temporal lobes of the brain.

Patch test: substance applied to the skin on a piece of gauze to determine its sensitivity to that substance. In this text, it refers to skin test for sensitivity to tuberculosis bacillus.

Pathogenic: causing disease.

Pediatrician: a specialist in the treatment of children's diseases.

Pediculosis: a skin disease produced by lice.

Pes planus: flat foot. (Seen recorded on physical examination charts as "P.P.").

Pellagra: a dietary deficiency disease of the skin and spinal cord.

Pleura: the membrane enveloping the lung and lining the internal surface of the chest cavity.

Pneumothorax: the presence of air or gas in the pleural cavity; it refers in this text to artificial pneumothorax produced by injecting air through a needle, causing collapse of the lung, thus allowing the lung to rest; used in treatment of pulmonary tuberculosis.

Prepsychotic: Pertaining to the mental state that precedes or is potentially capable of preceding a psychosis.

Prognosis: a prediction of the duration, course, and termination of a disease, based on all information available in the individual case and knowledge of how the disease behaves generally.

Projection: a mental mechanism by which a person indirectly conceals from himself his personal faults and socially disapproved motives by attributing them to others.

Psychiatry: the recognition and treatment of nervous disorders.

Psychoneurosis: term applied to a large group of functional disorders characterized by emotional states of anxiety and fear, and psychosomatic tension in different organs of the body.

Psychopath: a morally irresponsible person; one who continually comes into conflict with accepted behavior and the law.

Psychosis: major mental disorder involving profound thought, emotional, and personality disturbance that renders a person incapable of adequate self-management or adjustment to society.

Psychosomatic: of or pertaining to the mind and body; especially relating to a system of medicine which emphasizes the interdependence of mental processes and physical, or somatic, functions.

Puberty: the age at which the reproductive organs become functional.

Rapport: a harmonious counselor-client relationship, marked by the client's having confidence in the counselor.

Rationalization: a mental mechanism by which an individual justifies socially disapproved behavior by inventing "good and acceptable" reasons for the real reasons.

Retina: the light-receptive layer of the eye.

Rheumatic fever: a disease characterized by fever and painful arthritis that moves from joint to joint; often causes heart damage.

Riboflavin: Vitamin B2.

Rickets: a disease in children caused by a lack of vitamin D and resulting in poor bone formation.

Schizophrenia: a functional mental illness frequently terminating in mental regression; total withdrawal from reality into phantasies.

Scoliosis: abnormal lateral curvature of the spine.

Sebaceous gland: skin gland secreting oily material.

Self: includes everything which the individual experiences as part or characteristic of himself. It is the individual as known to the individual.

Sinus: air cavity in bone; usually refers to nasal sinus.

Sinusitis: inflammation of a sinus.

Somatic: pertaining to the body.

Spastic: characterized by a sudden muscular contraction.

Spirochete: a spiral-shaped microorganism.

Squint: see strabismus.

Staphylococcus: a round-shaped organism; often grows in groups resembling grapes.

Strabismus: a deviation of one of the eyes from its proper direction.

Streptococcus: a round-shaped organism that usually grows in chains.

Stye: an inflammation of the connective tissue of the eyelids near a hair follicle; hordeolum.

Subclinical: pertaining to a disease, the signs of which are so slight as to be unnoticeable; may not be demonstrable.

Sulfa drug: a drug of the sulfanilamide family, having marked power to arrest or hinder the growth of bacteria.

Synovial: pertaining to or secreting the fluid of a joint cavity.

Symptomatic: pertaining to a symptom.

Therapeutics: the science and art of healing.

Thiamin: vitamin B_1.

Thoracic: pertaining to the chest.

Trauma: injury or wound.

Trachoma: a contagious inflammation of the lining of the eyelid.

Tuberculin test: a skin test to determine tubercular infection.

Ulcer: an interruption of the continuity of a surface of the body with an inflamed base. (Gastric ulcer: ulcer of the lining of the stomach, etc.)

Urticaria: hives; a skin condition characterized by the appearance of intensely itching wheals.

Vaccination: inoculation with any organism to produce immunity against a given infectious disease.

Valvular insufficiency: imperfect closure of a heart valve.

Varicose veins: unnaturally swollen veins.

Ventricle: a small cavity or pouch; often refers to ventricle of heart: muscular chamber of the heart that pushes blood into the artery.

Vertigo: dizziness.

Virus: a group of disease-producing agents smaller than bacteria.

Vitamins: substances existing in minute quantities in natural foods and necessary for proper metabolism. Their absence produces deficiency diseases.

INDEX